SAUNDERS

VETERINARY ANATOMY
COLORING BOOK

EXPERT CONSULTANT

Baljit Singh, BVSc&AH, PhD

3M National Teaching Fellow
Professor
Department of Veterinary Biomedical Sciences
University of Saskatchewan
Saskatoon, Saskatchewan
Canada

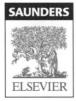

SAUNDERS

ELSEVIER

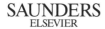

SAUNDERS
ELSEVIER

3251 Riverport Lane
Maryland Heights, Missouri 63043

SAUNDERS VETERINARY ANATOMY COLORING BOOK   978-1-4377-1439-5

Notice

Vice President and Publisher: Linda Duncan
Publisher: Penny Rudolph
Senior Developmental Editor: Shelly Stringer
Publishing Services Manager: Julie Eddy
Senior Project Manager: Celeste Clingan
Design Direction: Jessica Williams

Printed in United States

Last digit is the print number: 9 8 7 6 5 4 3 2

Working together to grow
libraries in developing countries

www.elsevier.com | www.bookaid.org | www.sabre.org

ELSEVIER   BOOK AID
              International   Sabre Foundation

ABOUT THE COLORING BOOK

Welcome to *Saunders Veterinary Anatomy Coloring Book!* With approximately 300 illustrations for you to study and color, the coloring book is designed to help you succeed in mastering veterinary anatomy. Whether you are a student of veterinary medicine or veterinary technology, this study tool will help you memorize the anatomy you need to know and give you a fun way to review the information you have studied. The interactive exercise of adding color to the images helps you learn and retain the anatomy of different body structures.

Saunders Veterinary Anatomy Coloring Book covers 🐕 canine, 🐈 feline, 🐴 equine, 🐖 porcine, 🐄 ruminant, and 🐦 avian anatomy, representing the range of species you need to know to be prepared to practice successfully. Each page includes a species-specific icon for easy identification of the species being covered. The book is divided into 7 regions of the body according to sections: The Head and Ventral Neck; The Neck, Back, and Vertebral Column; The Thorax; The Abdomen; The Pelvis and Reproductive Organs; The Forelimb; and The Hindlimb.

Saunders Veterinary Anatomy Coloring Book is an ideal companion for anyone studying veterinary anatomy. Use and review this book before an exam, before a class, or even before seeing your next patient.

How to Use The Book

Each page contains a brief statement describing the body part featured and its orientation view, followed by a crisp, easy-to-color illustration. Numbered lead lines clearly identify the structures to be colored and correspond to a numbered list appearing beneath the illustration. You can create your own "color code" by using the same color to fill in the boxed number appearing on the illustration, the anatomical structure, and the corresponding numbered box on the list below the illustration. An example of a completed illustration can be found on the inside front cover.

ILLUSTRATION CREDITS

Saunders Veterinary Anatomy Coloring Book includes black and white, two-dimensional versions of the line drawings as they appear in full color in Elsevier's well-established textbooks on anatomy:

- **Dyce, Sack, and Wensing:** *Textbook of Veterinary Anatomy*
- **Evans and de Lahunta:** *Guide to the Dissection of the Dog*
- **Evans and de Lahunta:** *Miller's Anatomy of the Dog*

CONTENTS

CONTENTS (CONT.)

Saunders Veterinary Anatomy Coloring Book
Copyright © 2011 by Saunders, an imprint of Elsevier Inc.

CONTENTS (CONT.)

CONTENTS (CONT.)

CONTENTS (CONT.)

CONTENTS (CONT.)

THE HEAD AND VENTRAL NECK

Figure 1-1   Lateral (*A*), dorsal (*B*), and ventral (*C*) views of the canine skull to show the extents of the cranial bones

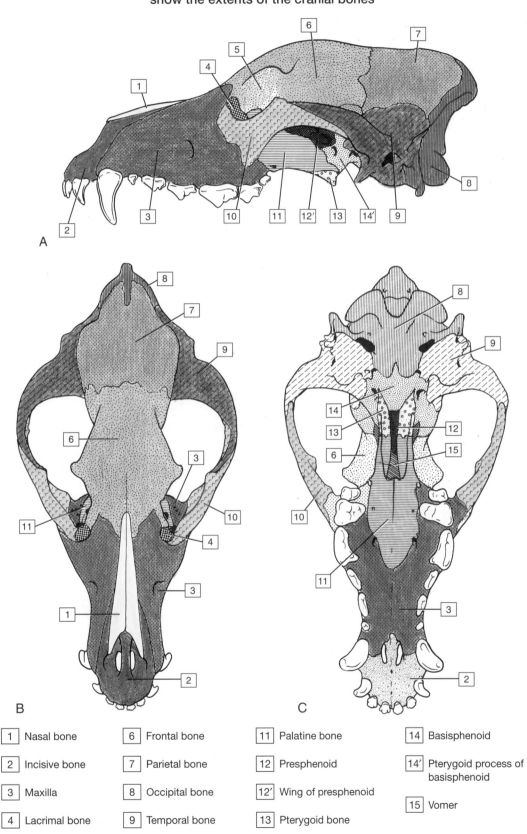

1	Nasal bone	6	Frontal bone	11	Palatine bone	14	Basisphenoid
2	Incisive bone	7	Parietal bone	12	Presphenoid	14′	Pterygoid process of basisphenoid
3	Maxilla	8	Occipital bone	12′	Wing of presphenoid		
4	Lacrimal bone	9	Temporal bone	13	Pterygoid bone	15	Vomer
5	Orbit	10	Zygomatic bone				

Figure 1-2 Dorsal view of the canine skull

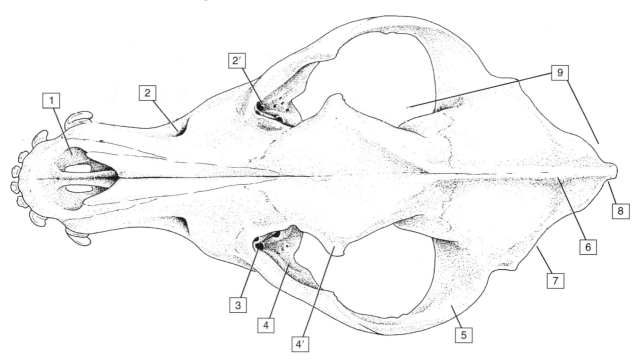

1 Nasal aperture	5 Zygomatic arch
2 Infraorbital foramen	6 External sagittal crest
2' Maxillary foramen	7 Nuchal crest
3 Fossa for lacrimal sac	8 External occipital protuberance
4 Orbit	9 Cranium
4' Zygomatic process of frontal bone	

Figure 1-3   Ventral view of the canine skull

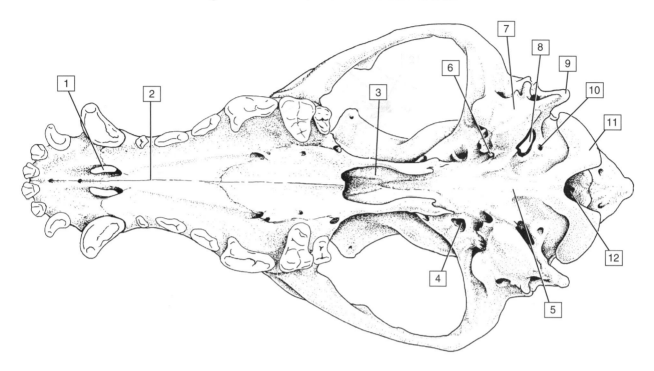

1	Palatine fissure	7	Tympanic bulla
2	Hard palate	8	Jugular foramen
3	Choanal region	9	Paracondylar process
4	Oval foramen	10	Hypoglossal canal
5	Base of cranium	11	Occipital condyle
6	Foramen lacerum	12	Foramen magnum

Figure 1-4   Hyoid apparatus and larynx suspended from the temporal region
of a canine skull

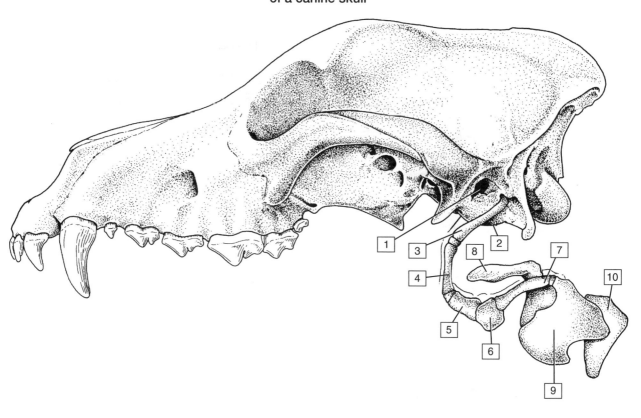

1	External acoustic meatus	6	Basihyoid
2	Tympanic bulla	7	Thyrohyoid
3	Stylohyoid	8	Epiglottic cartilage
4	Epihyoid	9	Thyroid cartilage
5	Ceratohyoid	10	Cricoid cartilage

Figure 1-5   Canine oral cavity and tongue

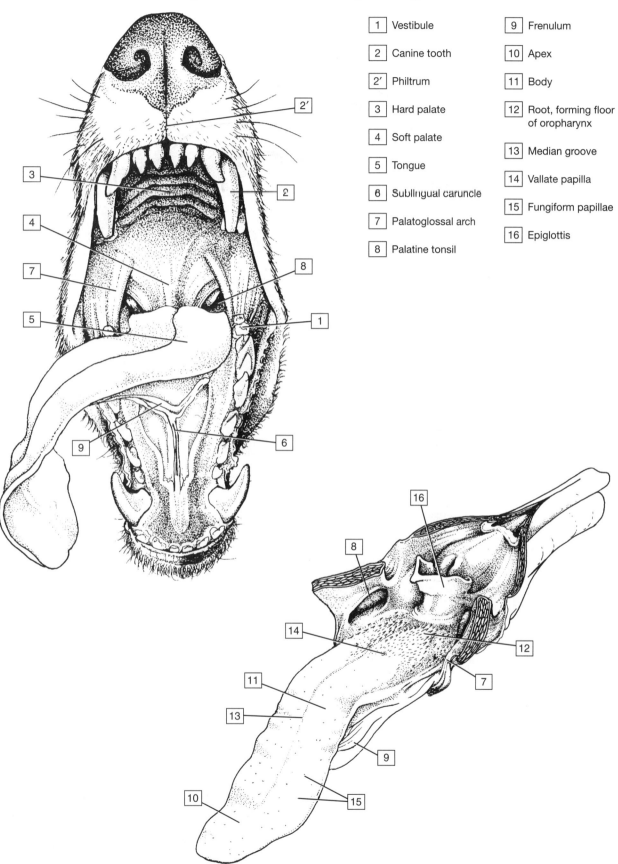

1	Vestibule	9	Frenulum
2	Canine tooth	10	Apex
2′	Philtrum	11	Body
3	Hard palate	12	Root, forming floor of oropharynx
4	Soft palate	13	Median groove
5	Tongue	14	Vallate papilla
6	Sublingual caruncle	15	Fungiform papillae
7	Palatoglossal arch	16	Epiglottis
8	Palatine tonsil		

Figure 1-6   Muscles of the canine tongue and pharynx

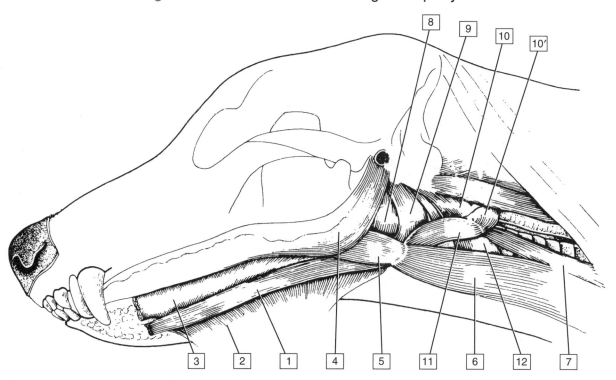

1	Gleniohyoideus	8	Hyopharyngeus (two parts)
2	Mylohyoideus	9	Hyopharyngeus (two parts)
3	Genioglossus	10	Thyropharyngeus
4	Styloglossus	10′	Cricopharyngeus
5	Hyoglossus	11	Thyrohyoideus
6	Sternohyoideus	12	Cricothyroideus
7	Sternothyroideus		

Figure 1-7   Canine salivary glands

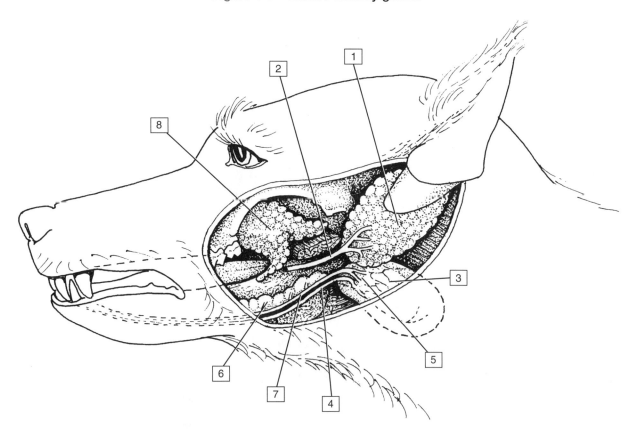

1 Parotid gland	5 Caudal part of compact sublingual gland
2 Parotid duct	6 Rostral part of compact sublingual gland
3 Mandibular gland	7 Major sublingual duct
4 Mandibular duct	8 Zygomatic gland

**Figure 1-8 Canine simple tooth and muscles of mastication,
left lateral aspect**

1 Enamel

2 Dentine

3 Cement

4 Pulp

5 Apical foramen

6 Periodontal ligament

7 Socket (alveolus)

8 Gum

9 Temporalis

10 Masseter

11 Rostral and belly of digastricus

12 Mylohyoideus

13 Medial pterygoid

14 Origin of lateral pterygoid

15 Tongue

16 Mandible

17 Zygomatic arch

18 Level of transection

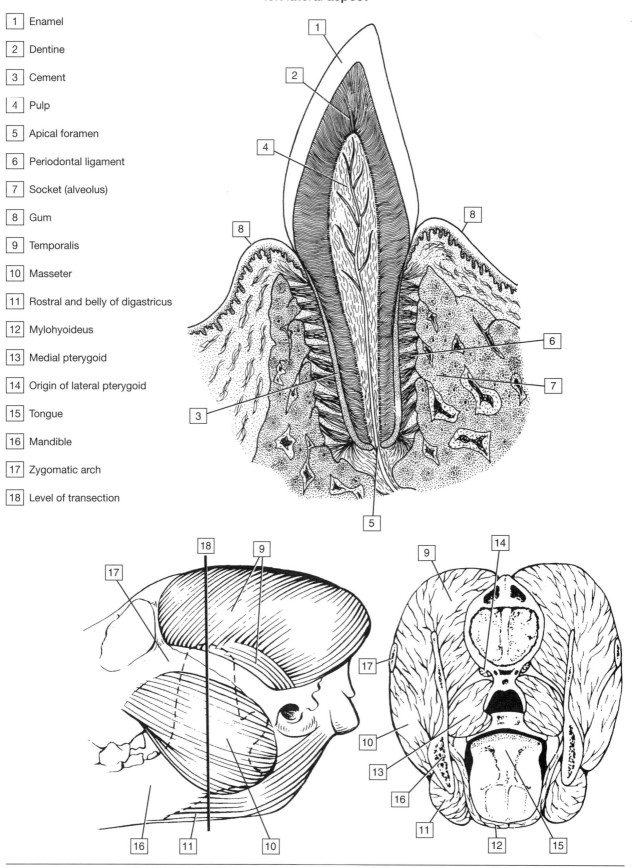

Figure 1-9 **Development of canine dental plate and enamel organ**

A, Development of canine dental plate and, *B, C,* enamel organ. *D,* Deciduous tooth before eruption.

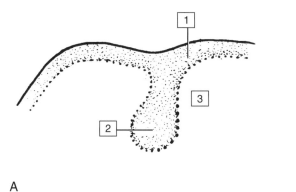

A

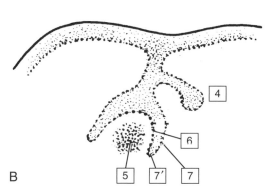

B

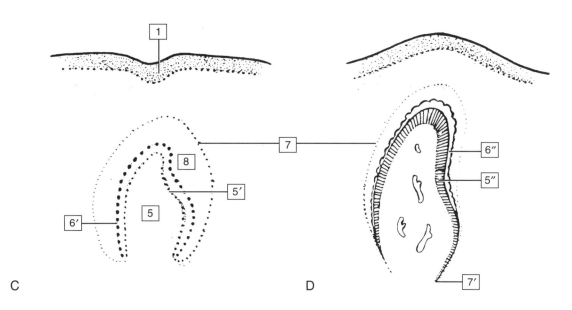

C

D

1	Epithelium of oral cavity	6	Inner dental epithelium (future ameloblasts)
2	Dental plate	6′	Ameloblasts
3	Mesenchyme	6″	Enamel
4	Bud of a permanent tooth	7	Outer dental epithelium
5	Dental papilla	7′	Transition of inner and outer dental epithelia (where root formation occurs)
5′	Odontoblasts (differentiated from the outer cell layer of the papilla)	8	Enamel reticulum
5″	Dentine		

Figure 1-10   Transverse section of the canine larynx

Arrows on the left: action of cricoarytenoideus lateralis on arytenoid cartilage.
Arrows on the right: action of cricoarytenoideus dorsalis on arytenoid cartilage.

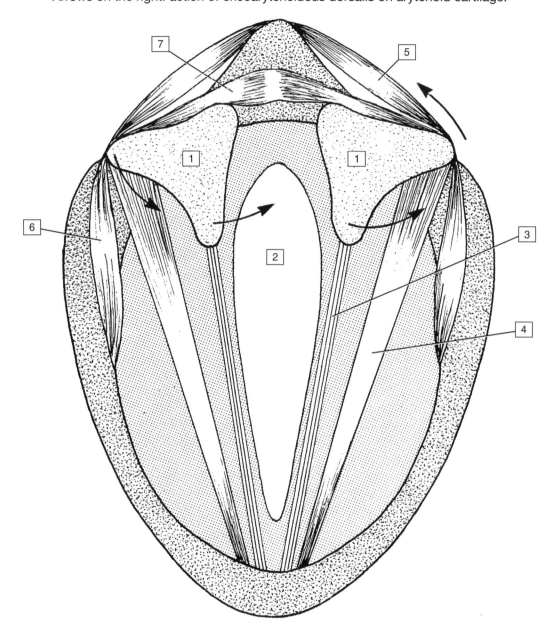

1	Location of the cricoarytenoid joint	5	Cricoarytenoideus dorsalis
2	Glottic cleft	6	Cricoarytenoideus lateralis
3	Vocal ligament in vocal fold	7	Arytenoideus transversus
4	Thyroarytenoideus		

Figure 1-11   Organization of the canine brain-pituitary-peripheral organ axis

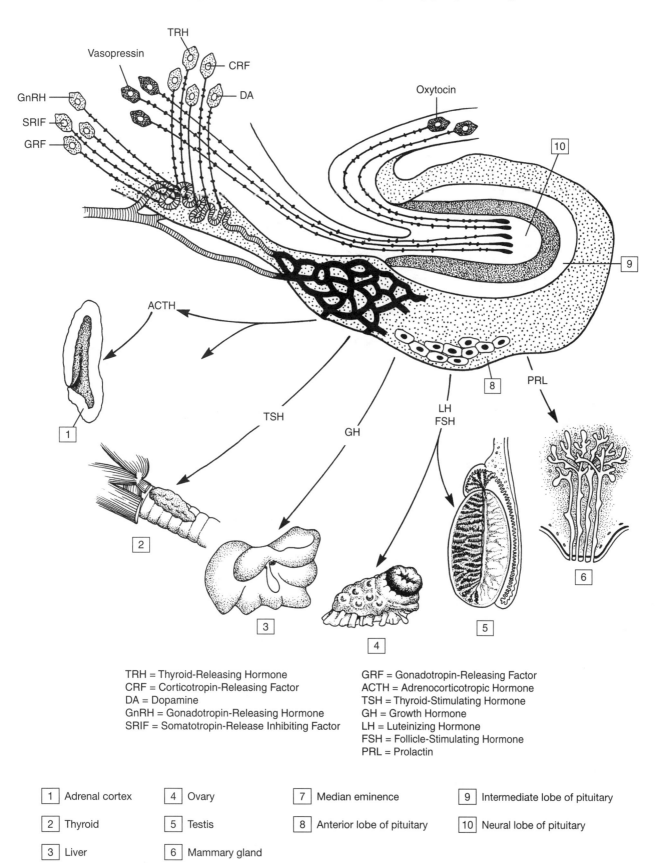

TRH = Thyroid-Releasing Hormone
CRF = Corticotropin-Releasing Factor
DA = Dopamine
GnRH = Gonadotropin-Releasing Hormone
SRIF = Somatotropin-Release Inhibiting Factor

GRF = Gonadotropin-Releasing Factor
ACTH = Adrenocorticotropic Hormone
TSH = Thyroid-Stimulating Hormone
GH = Growth Hormone
LH = Luteinizing Hormone
FSH = Follicle-Stimulating Hormone
PRL = Prolactin

1 Adrenal cortex	4 Ovary	7 Median eminence	9 Intermediate lobe of pituitary
2 Thyroid	5 Testis	8 Anterior lobe of pituitary	10 Neural lobe of pituitary
3 Liver	6 Mammary gland		

Figure 1-12   Arteries of the canine head

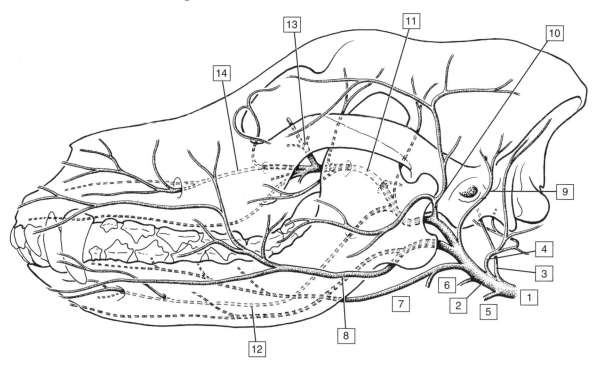

1	Common carotid a.	8	Facial a.
2	External carotid a.	9	Caudal auricular a.
3	Internal carotid a.	10	Superficial temporal a.
4	Occipital a.	11	Maxillary a.
5	Cranial laryngeal a.	12	Inferior alveolar a.
6	Ascending pharyngeal a.	13	External ophthalmic a.
7	Lingual a.	14	Infraorbital a.

Figure 1-13   Lymph drainage of the canine head, neck, and mammary glands

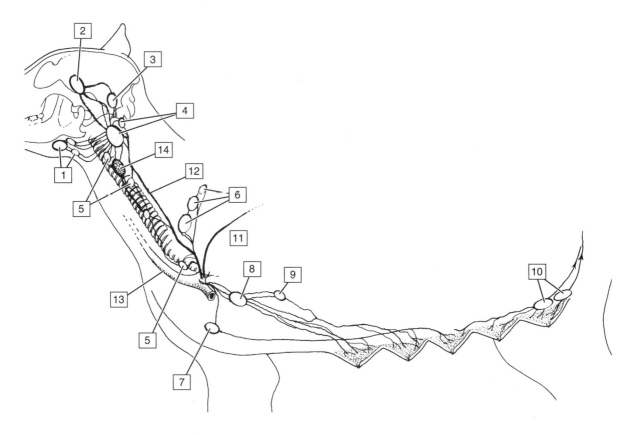

1 Mandibular nodes	8 Axillary node
2 Parotid node	9 Accessory axillary node
3 Lateral retropharyngeal node	10 Superficial inguinal nodes
4 Medial retropharyngeal nodes	11 Thoracic duct
5 Cranial and caudal deep cervical nodes	12 Tracheal duct
6 Superficial cervical nodes	13 External jugular vein
7 Sternal node	14 Thyroid gland

Figure 1-14   Canine reflex chain in which an interneuron is interposed

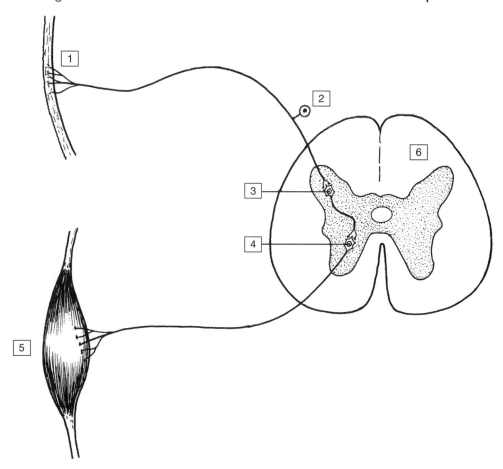

1	Skin receptor	4	Synapse at efferent neuron
2	Afferent neuron	5	Muscle
3	Synapse at interneuron	6	Spinal cord

Figure 1-15   The course of fibers within the canine spinal cord

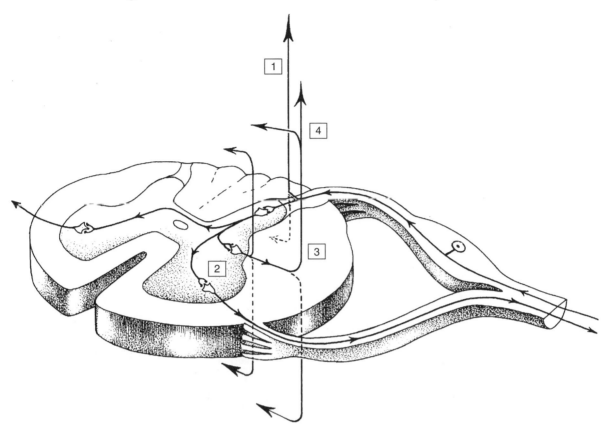

1 Afferent fibers in the dorsal funiculus travelling toward the brain (others end on interneurons in the dorsal horn)	**3** Impulses transmitted to other interneurons transmitting impulses caudally or cranially within the spinal cord
2 Impulses transmitted directly to efferent neurons	**4** Impulses extending to the brain

Figure 1-16 Dorsal view of the canine brain

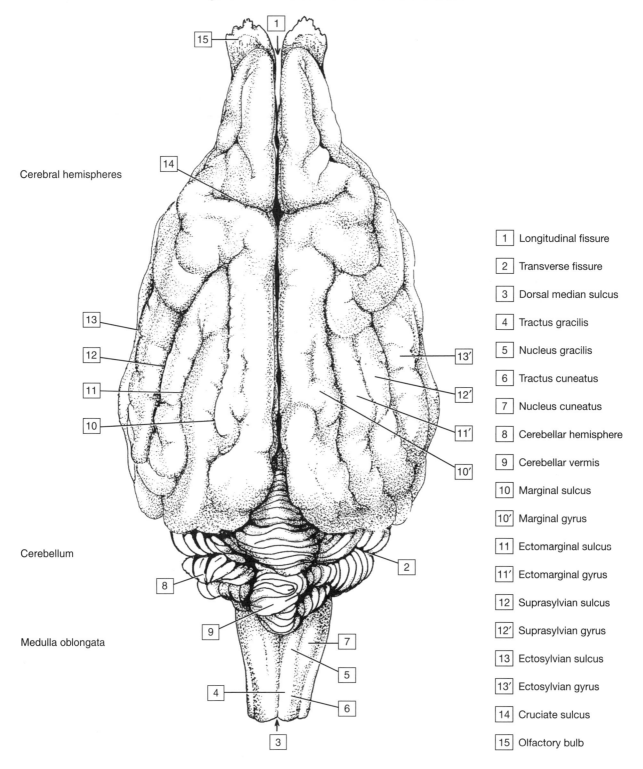

Cerebral hemispheres

Cerebellum

Medulla oblongata

1	Longitudinal fissure
2	Transverse fissure
3	Dorsal median sulcus
4	Tractus gracilis
5	Nucleus gracilis
6	Tractus cuneatus
7	Nucleus cuneatus
8	Cerebellar hemisphere
9	Cerebellar vermis
10	Marginal sulcus
10'	Marginal gyrus
11	Ectomarginal sulcus
11'	Ectomarginal gyrus
12	Suprasylvian sulcus
12'	Suprasylvian gyrus
13	Ectosylvian sulcus
13'	Ectosylvian gyrus
14	Cruciate sulcus
15	Olfactory bulb

Figure 1-17   Ventral view of the canine brain

I-XII designate the appropriate cranial nerves.

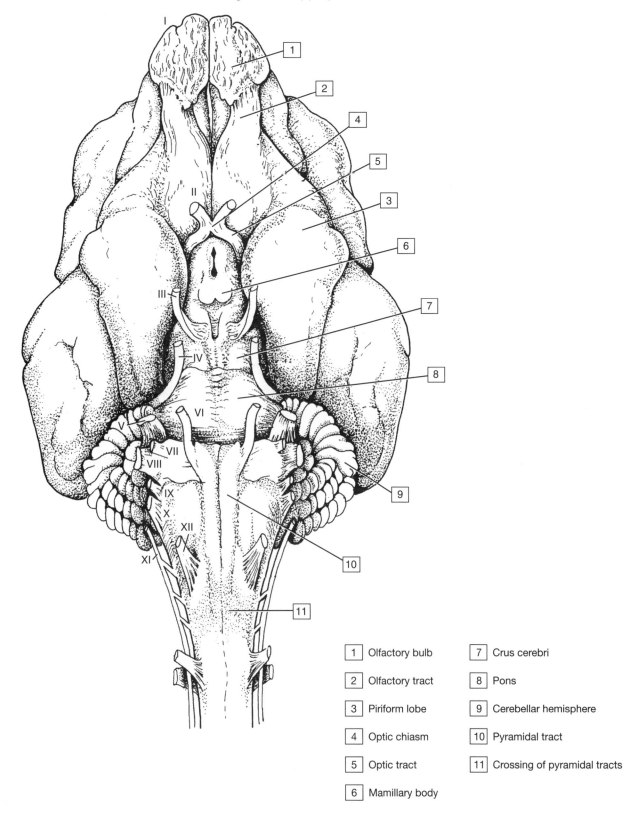

1	Olfactory bulb	7	Crus cerebri
2	Olfactory tract	8	Pons
3	Piriform lobe	9	Cerebellar hemisphere
4	Optic chiasm	10	Pyramidal tract
5	Optic tract	11	Crossing of pyramidal tracts
6	Mamillary body		

Figure 1-18   Median section of the canine brain

Part of the medial wall of the hemisphere has been removed.

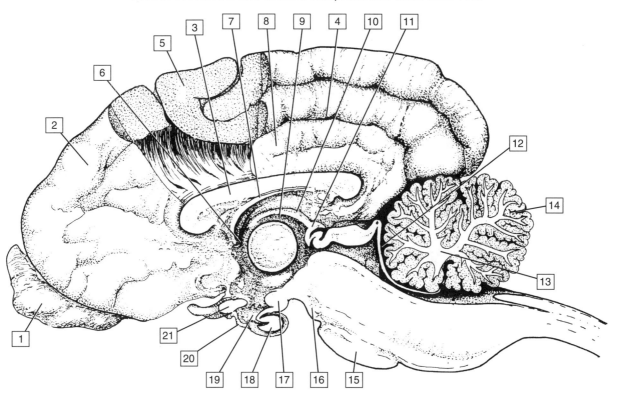

1	Olfactory bulb	12	Rostral medullary velum
2	Hemisphere	13	Corpus medullare
3	Corpus callosum	14	Cerebellar cortex
4	Splenial sulcus	15	Pons
5	Cerebral cortex	16	Crus cerebri
6	Interventricular foramen	17	Mamillary body
7	Fornix	18	Hypophysis
8	Cingulate gyrus	19	Infundibulum
9	Thalamus	20	Tuber cinereum
10	Epithalamus	21	Optic chiasm
11	Epiphysis		

Figure 1-19 Canine brainstem showing the nuclei in an adult mammal

Roman numerals are used for nuclei of some cranial nerves.
A = afferent nuclei; B = efferent nuclei.

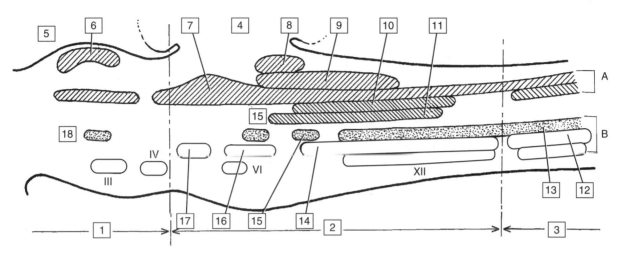

1	Mesencephalon	
2	Rhombencephalon	
3	Spinal cord	
4	Cerebellum	
5	Tectum mesencephali	
6	Rostral colliculus (SSA)	
7	Trigeminal nuclei (SA)	
8	Cochlear nuclei (SSA)	
9	Vestibular nuclei (SSA)	
10	Solitary nucleus of VII, IX, X (VA)	
11	Gustatory nuclei of VII, IX (SVA)	
12	Motor nucleus of XI (GSE)	
13	Motor nucleus of X (GVE)	
14	Nucleus ambiguous of IX, X (GSE)	
15	Salivatory nuclei of VII, IX (GVE)	
16	Motor nucleus of VII (GSE)	
17	Motor nucleus of V (GSE)	
18	Parasympathetic nucleus of III (GVE)	

Figure 1-20   A simplified schema of the canine visual and pupillary reflex
pathways

Thick lines, special somatic visual fibers; *thin lines,* sympathetic fibers; *broken
lines,* parasympathetic fibers.

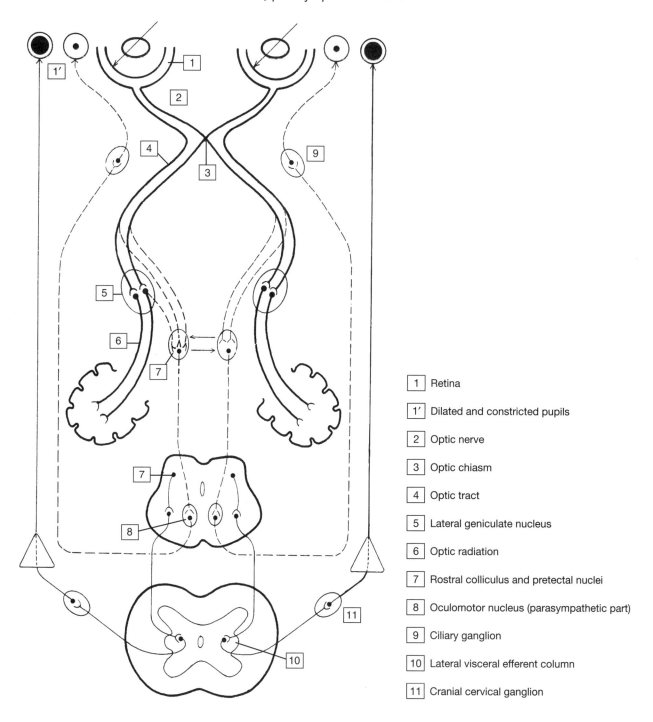

1	Retina
1′	Dilated and constricted pupils
2	Optic nerve
3	Optic chiasm
4	Optic tract
5	Lateral geniculate nucleus
6	Optic radiation
7	Rostral colliculus and pretectal nuclei
8	Oculomotor nucleus (parasympathetic part)
9	Ciliary ganglion
10	Lateral visceral efferent column
11	Cranial cervical ganglion

Figure 1-21   Relay diagram of the pyramidal (*continuous line*) and the extrapyramidal (*interrupted line*) systems

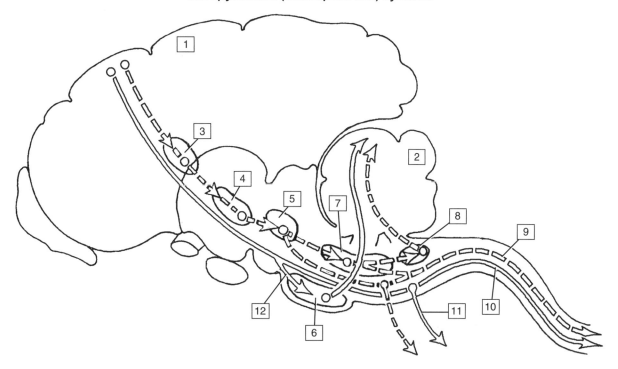

1	Motor cortex	7	Reticular formation
2	Cerebellum	8	Olivary nucleus
3	Basal nuclei	9	Rubrospinal tract
4	Substantia nigra (mesencephalon)	10	Corticospinal fibers
5	Red nucleus (mesencephalon)	11	Corticobulbar fibers
6	Pontine nuclei (metencephalon)	12	Corticopontine fibers

Figure 1-22   Arteries on the ventral surface of the canine brain

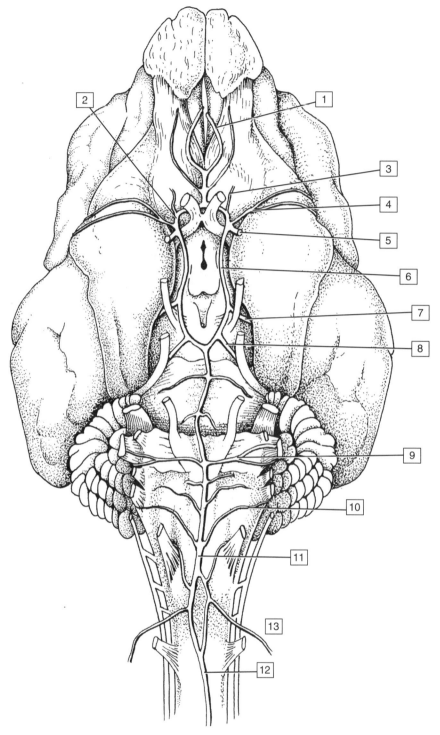

1	Internal ethmoidal a.
2	Rostral cerebral a.
3	Internal ophthalmic a.
4	Middle cerebral a.
5	Internal carotid a.
6	Caudal communicating a.
7	Caudal cerebral a.
8	Rostral cerebellar a.
9	Labyrinthine a.
10	Caudal cerebellar a.
11	Basilar a.
12	Ventral spinal a.
13	Vertebral a.

Figure 1-23   Distribution pattern of the canine facial nerve

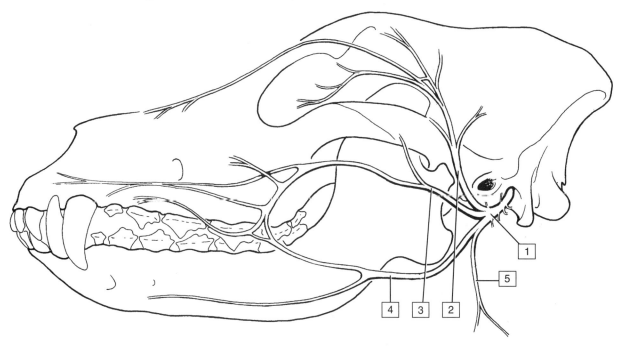

1	Facial n.
2	Auriculopalpebral n.
3	Dorsal buccal branch
4	Ventral buccal branch
5	Cervical branch

Figure 1-24 Canine eye opened to show the three tunics, which have been drawn thicker than they actually are

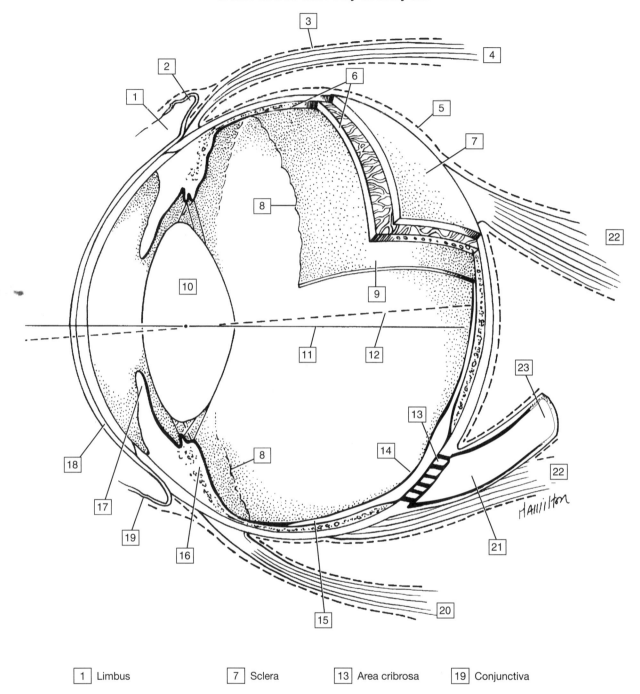

1	Limbus	7	Sclera	13	Area cribrosa	19	Conjunctiva

1	Limbus
2	Upper fornix
3	Deep muscular fascia
4	Dorsal rectus muscle
5	Vagina bulbi
6	Choroid

7	Sclera
8	Ora serrata
9	Retina
10	Lens
11	Optic axis
12	Visual axis

13	Area cribrosa
14	Optic disc
15	Retina
16	Ciliary body
17	Iris
18	Cornea

19	Conjunctiva
20	Ventral rectus muscle
21	Optic nerve
22	Retractor bulbi
23	Sheath of optic nerve

Figure 1-25   Anterior part of the canine eye in section

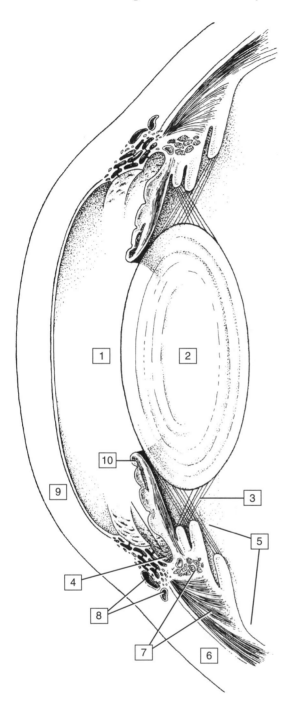

1	Anterior chamber
2	Lens
3	Zonular fibers
4	Iridocorneal angle
5	Ciliary body
6	Sclera
7	Ciliary muscles
8	Venous plexus of sclera
9	Cornea
10	Iris with the sphincter and dilator muscles shown

Figure 1-26   Stumps of canine ocular muscles viewed from behind
the left eyeball

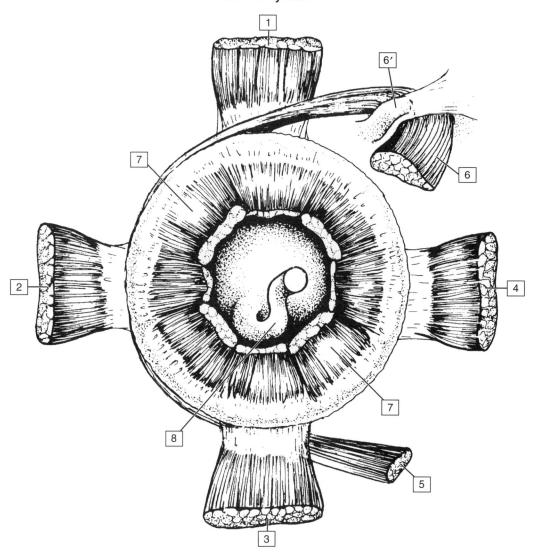

1	Dorsal rectus m.		6	Dorsal oblique m.
2	Lateral rectus m.		6'	Trochlea
3	Ventral rectus m.		7	Retractor bulbi
4	Medial rectus m.		8	Optic nerve
5	Ventral oblique m.			

Figure 1-27   Canine sensory nerve endings of the skin

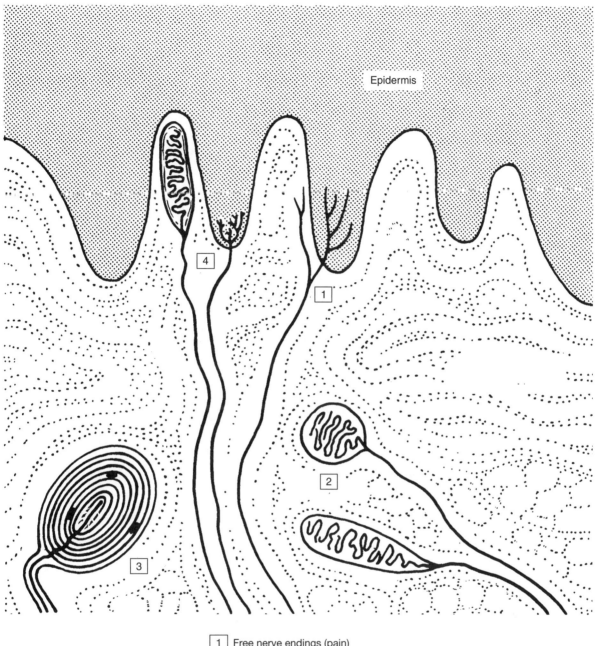

1	Free nerve endings (pain)
2	Bulbous corpuscles (heat or cold)
3	Lamellar corpuscles (vibration)
4	Meniscoid nerve endings (touch)

Figure 1-28   Canine hair follicle with accessory structures

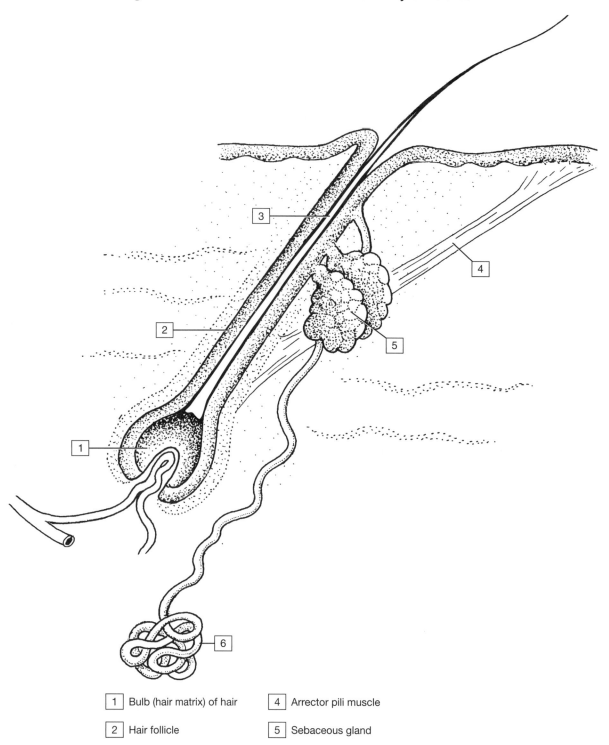

1	Bulb (hair matrix) of hair	4	Arrector pili muscle
2	Hair follicle	5	Sebaceous gland
3	Root of hair	6	Sweat gland. In the adult, many glands open independently, not into hair follicles.

Figure 1-29   Superficial dissection of the canine head

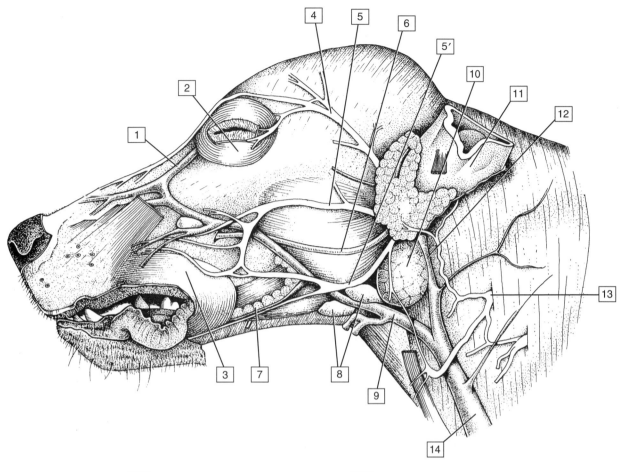

1 Angularis oculi vein	**8** Mandibular lymph nodes
2 Orbicularis oculi	**9** Linguofacial vein
3 Orbicularis oris	**10** Mandibular gland
4 Auriculopalpebral nerve	**11** Base of ear
5 Dorsal buccal branch of facial nerve	**12** Maxillary vein
5′ Ventral buccal branch of facial nerve	**13** Second cervical nerve
6 Parotid duct	**14** External jugular vein
7 Buccal salivary glands	

Figure 1-30   Dissection of the canine orbit and ptergopalatine fossa, lateral view

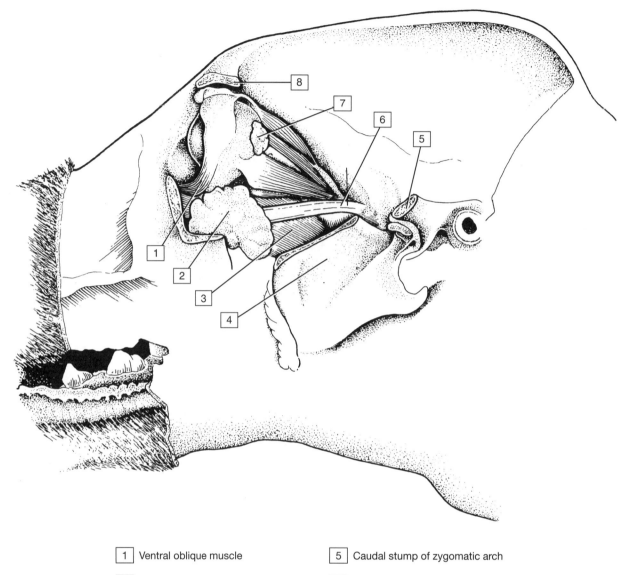

1	Ventral oblique muscle	5	Caudal stump of zygomatic arch
2	Zygomatic gland	6	Maxillary nerve
3	Medial pterygoid muscle	7	Lacrimal gland
4	Coronoid process of mandible, cut	8	Zygomatic process of frontal bone

Figure 1-31   The major arteries (gray) and veins (white) of the canine head. The ramus of the mandible has been removed.

The major arteries (*gray*) and veins (*black*) of the canine head. The ramus of the mandible has been removed.

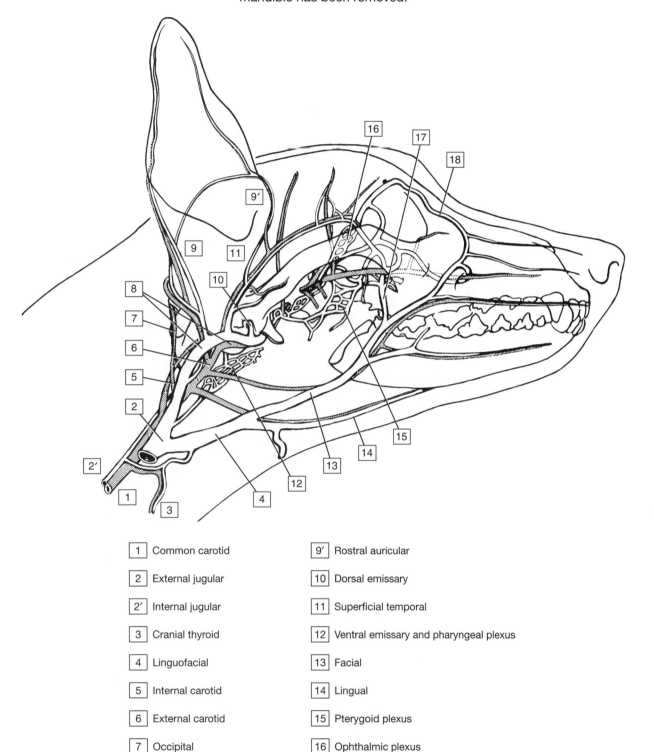

1	Common carotid	9′	Rostral auricular
2	External jugular	10	Dorsal emissary
2′	Internal jugular	11	Superficial temporal
3	Cranial thyroid	12	Ventral emissary and pharyngeal plexus
4	Linguofacial	13	Facial
5	Internal carotid	14	Lingual
6	External carotid	15	Pterygoid plexus
7	Occipital	16	Ophthalmic plexus
8	Maxillary	17	Deep facial
9	Caudal auricular	18	Angularis oculi

Figure 1-32   Transverse section of the canine neck at the level of the fifth
cervical vertebra

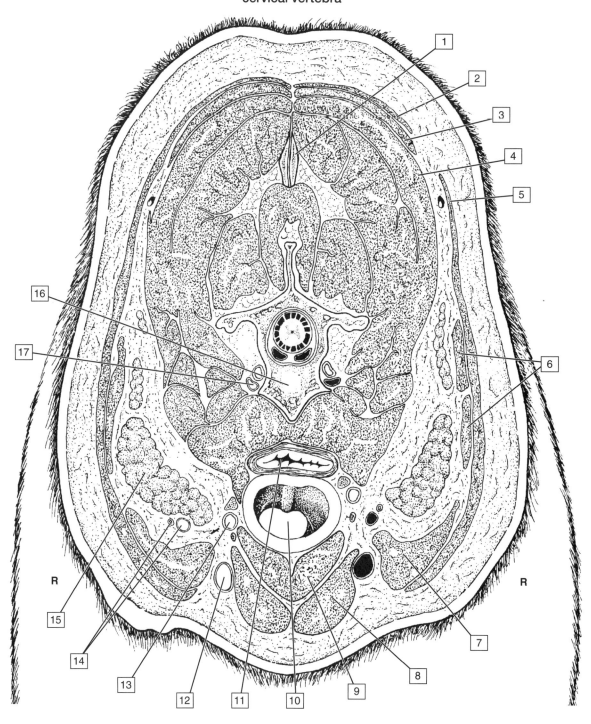

1 Nuchal ligament	6 Omotransversarius	11 Esophagus	15 Superficial cervical lymph nodes
2 Trapezius	7 Cleidomastoideus	12 External jugular vein	16 Fifth cervical vertebra
3 Rhomboideus	8 Sternocephalicus	13 Common carotid artery, vagosympathetic trunk, and recurrent laryngeal nerve	17 Vertebral vessels
4 Splenius	9 Sternothyrohyoideus		
5 Cleidocervicalis	10 Trachea	14 Superficial cervical vessels	

Figure 1-33   Lymphatic structures of the canine head and neck

The inset shows the approximate areas of drainage of the principal nodes.

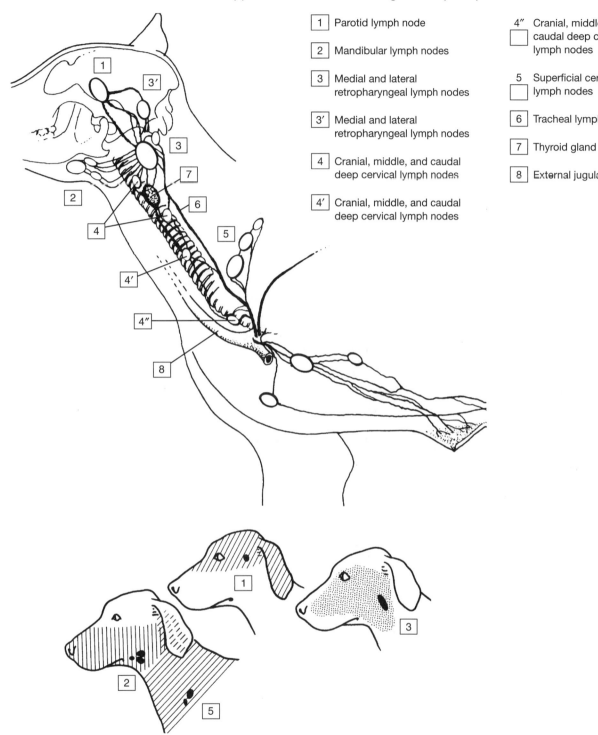

1 Parotid lymph node

2 Mandibular lymph nodes

3 Medial and lateral retropharyngeal lymph nodes

3' Medial and lateral retropharyngeal lymph nodes

4 Cranial, middle, and caudal deep cervical lymph nodes

4' Cranial, middle, and caudal deep cervical lymph nodes

4" Cranial, middle, and caudal deep cervical lymph nodes

5 Superficial cervical lymph nodes

6 Tracheal lymph trunk

7 Thyroid gland

8 External jugular vein

Figure 1-34   Superficial nerves of the canine neck, lateral aspect

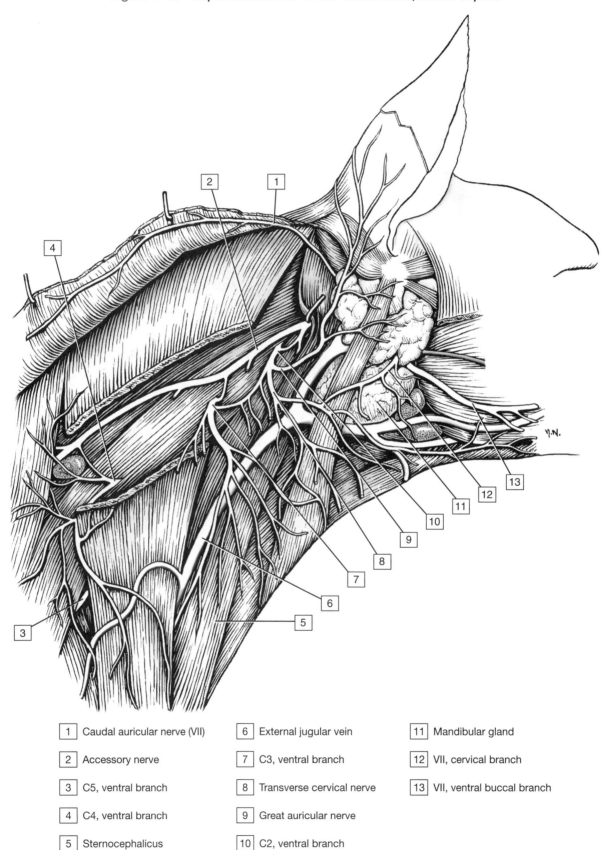

1	Caudal auricular nerve (VII)	6	External jugular vein	11	Mandibular gland
2	Accessory nerve	7	C3, ventral branch	12	VII, cervical branch
3	C5, ventral branch	8	Transverse cervical nerve	13	VII, ventral buccal branch
4	C4, ventral branch	9	Great auricular nerve		
5	Sternocephalicus	10	C2, ventral branch		

Figure 1-35 Veins of the canine neck, ventral aspect

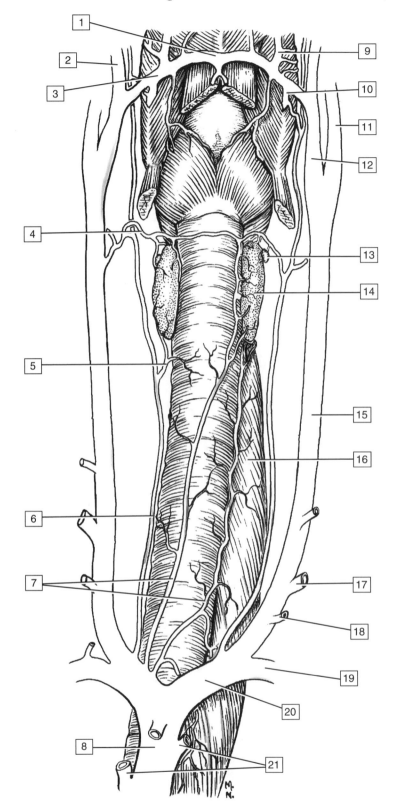

1	Hyoid venous arch
2	Facial
3	Lingual
4	Cranial thyroid
5	Middle thyroid
6	Right internal jugular
7	Caudal thyroid veins
8	Cranial vena cava
9	Lingual
10	Cranial laryngeal
11	Maxillary
12	Linguofacial
13	Parathyroid gland
14	Thyroid gland
15	External jugular
16	Esophagus
17	Superficial cervical
18	Cephalic
19	Subclavian
20	Brachiocephalic
21	Costocervical veins

Figure 1-36   Disarticulated puppy skull, ventral view

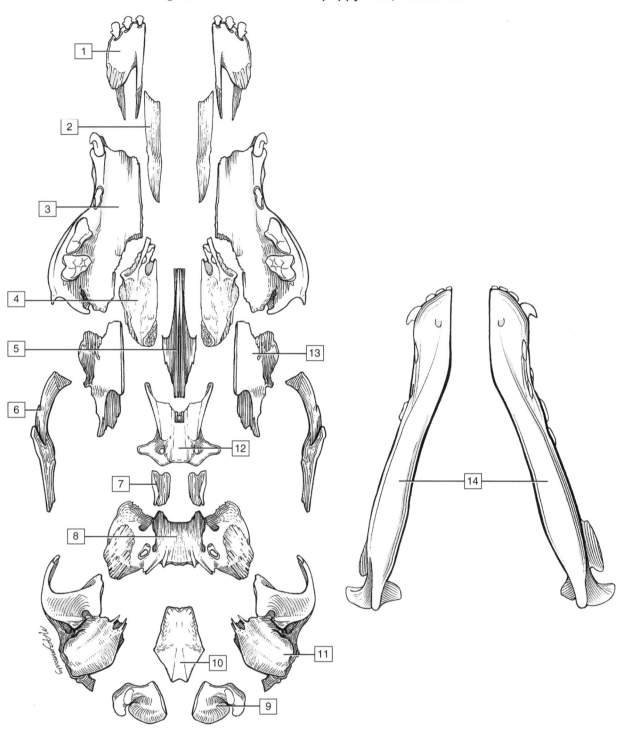

1	Incisive	5	Vomer	9	Exoccipital	13	Palatine
2	Nasal	6	Zygomatic	10	Basioccipital	14	Mandible
3	Maxilla	7	Pterygoid	11	Temporal		
4	Ethmoid	8	Basisphenoid	12	Presphenoid		

Saunders Veterinary Anatomy Coloring Book

Figure 1-37   Muscles of the canine pharynx and tongue, left lateral view, left mandible removed

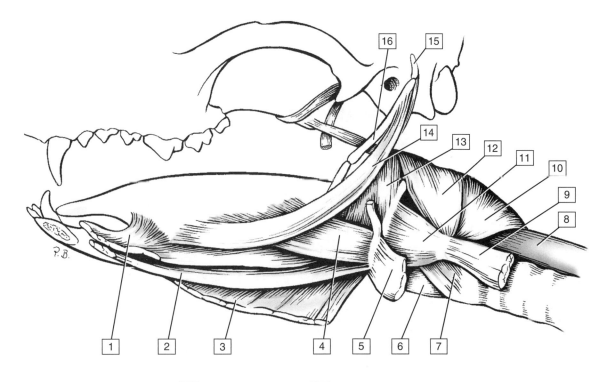

1	Genioglossus	9	Sternothyroideus
2	Geniohyoideus	10	Cricopharyngeus
3	Mylohyoideus	11	Thyrohyoideus
4	Hypoglossus	12	Thyropharyngeus
5	Sternohyoideus	13	Hyopharyngeus
6	Thyroid cartilage	14	Styloglossus
7	Cricothyroideus	15	Tympanohyoid cartilage
8	Esophagus	16	Stylohyoid bone

Figure 1-38   Canine extrinsic ocular muscles and their action on the left eyeball

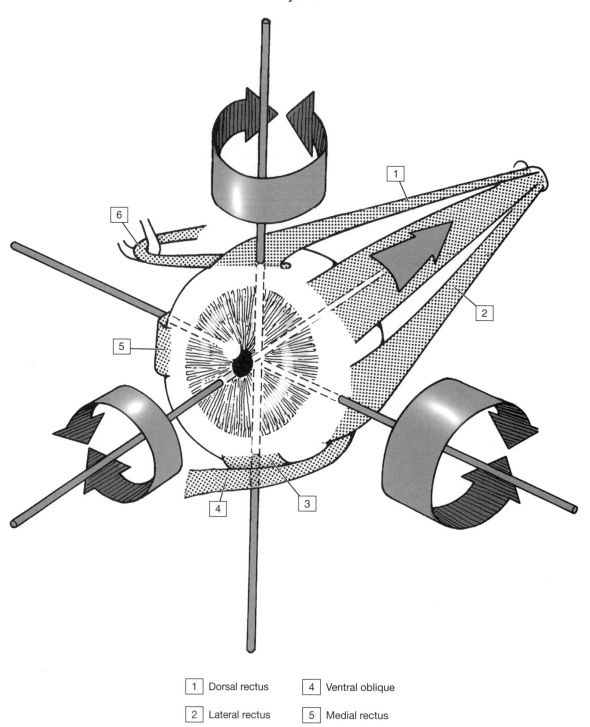

1	Dorsal rectus	4	Ventral oblique
2	Lateral rectus	5	Medial rectus
3	Ventral rectus	6	Dorsal oblique

THE HEAD AND VENTRAL NECK 1

Figure 1-39   Superficial branches of the canine facial and trigeminal nerves

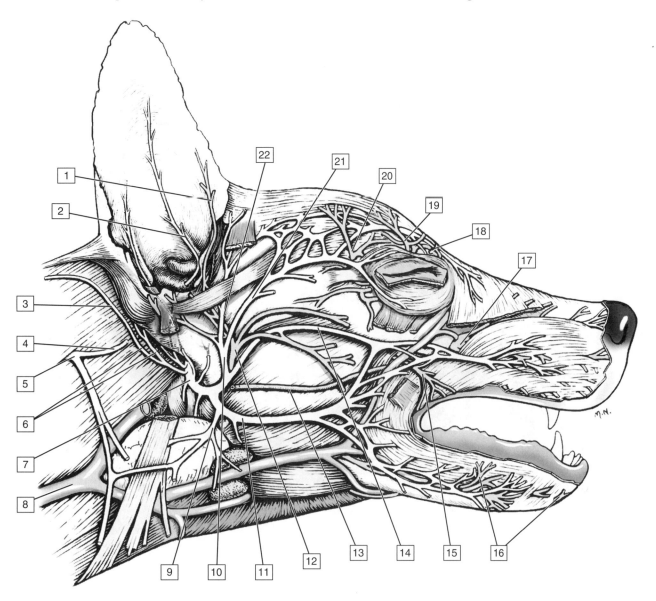

1 Rostral auricular nerve	9 Cervical branch	17 Infraorbital nerve
2 Internal auricular branch	10 Auriculopalpebral nerve	18 Infratrochlear nerve
3 Caudal auricular branch to platysma	11 Ventral buccal branch	19 Frontal nerve
4 Great auricular nerve	12 Auriculotemporal nerve V	20 Zygomaticotemporal nerve
5 C2, ventral branch	13 Parotid duct (cut)	21 Palpebral nerve
6 Caudal auricular branches	14 Dorsal buccal branch	22 Rostral auricular nerve
7 Facial nerve VII	15 Buccalis nerve	
8 External jugular vein	16 Mental nerves	

Figure 1-40   Branches of canine common carotid artery, superficial lateral view, part of digastricus removed

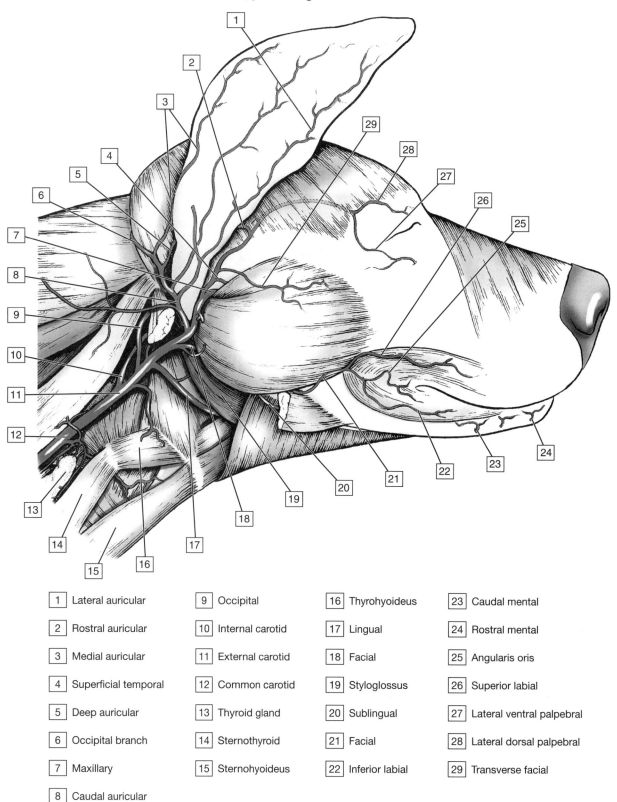

1 Lateral auricular	9 Occipital	16 Thyrohyoideus	23 Caudal mental
2 Rostral auricular	10 Internal carotid	17 Lingual	24 Rostral mental
3 Medial auricular	11 External carotid	18 Facial	25 Angularis oris
4 Superficial temporal	12 Common carotid	19 Styloglossus	26 Superior labial
5 Deep auricular	13 Thyroid gland	20 Sublingual	27 Lateral ventral palpebral
6 Occipital branch	14 Sternothyroid	21 Facial	28 Lateral dorsal palpebral
7 Maxillary	15 Sternohyoideus	22 Inferior labial	29 Transverse facial
8 Caudal auricular			

Figure 1-41   Canine muscles, nerves, and salivary glands medial to right
mandible, lateral view

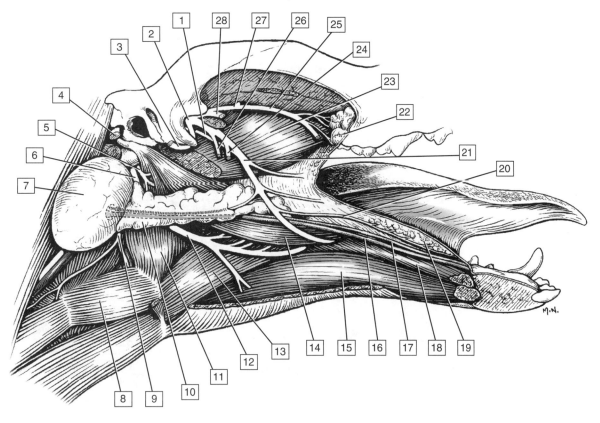

1	Chorda tympani
2	Mandibular branch of V
3	Auriculotemporal nerve
4	Facial nerve
5	Glossopharyngeal nerve
6	Hypoglossal nerve
7	Mandibular gland
8	Thyrohyoideus
9	Cranial laryngeal nerve
10	Monostomatic sublingual gland
11	Hyopharyngeus
12	Hypoglossal nerve
13	Hypoglossus
14	Styloglossus
15	Geniohyoideus
16	Mandibular duct
17	Sublingual duct
18	Genioglossus
19	Polystomatic sublingual gland
20	Sublingual nerve
21	Lingual nerve
22	Zygomatic gland
23	Medial pterygoid
24	Inferior alveolar nerve
25	Buccal nerve
26	Mylohyoid nerve
27	Deep temporal branch
28	Masseteric nerve

Figure 1-42   Meninges and ventricles of the canine brain, median plane

Arrows indicate flow of cerebrospinal fluid.

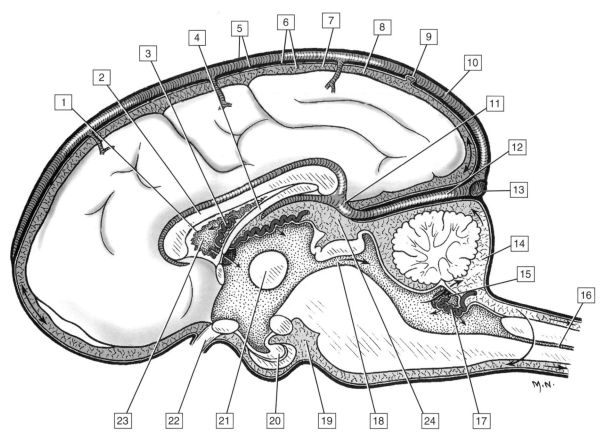

1 Cut edge of septum pellucidum	13 Transverse sinus
2 Corpus callosum	14 Cerebellomedullary cistern
3 Choroid plexus, lateral ventricle	15 Lateral aperture of fourth ventricle
4 Fornix of hippocampus	16 Central canal
5 Dura	17 Choroid plexus, fourth ventricle
6 Arachnoid membrane and trabeculae	18 Mesencephalic aqueduct
7 Subarachnoid space	19 Intercrural cistern
8 Pia	20 Neurohypophysis
9 Arachnoid villus	21 Interthalamic adhesion
10 Dorsal sagittal sinus	22 Optic nerve
11 Great cerebral vein	23 Lateral ventricle over caudate nucleus
12 Straight sinus	24 Quadrigeminal cistern

Figure 1-43 Ventral view of the canine brain, cranial nerves, and brain stem

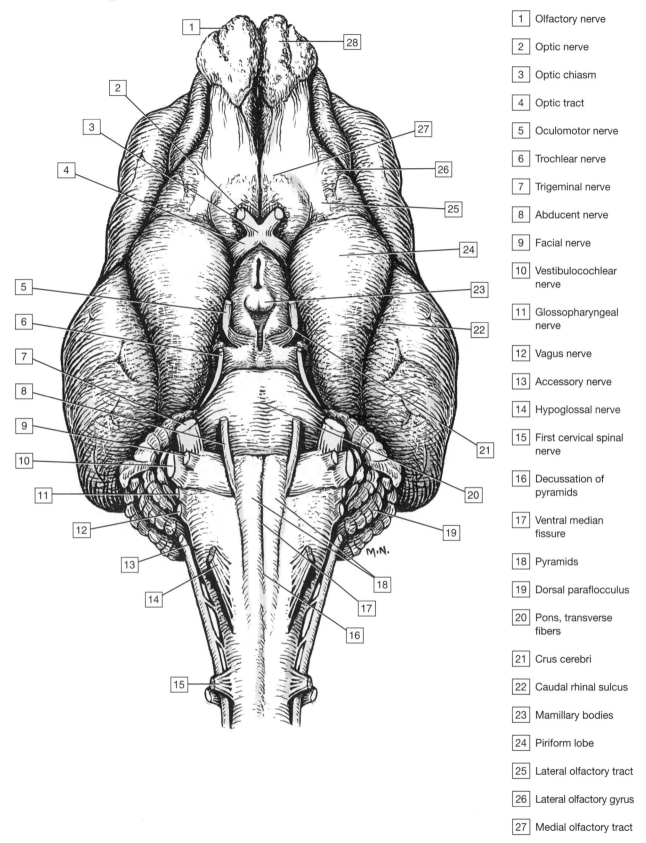

1	Olfactory nerve
2	Optic nerve
3	Optic chiasm
4	Optic tract
5	Oculomotor nerve
6	Trochlear nerve
7	Trigeminal nerve
8	Abducent nerve
9	Facial nerve
10	Vestibulocochlear nerve
11	Glossopharyngeal nerve
12	Vagus nerve
13	Accessory nerve
14	Hypoglossal nerve
15	First cervical spinal nerve
16	Decussation of pyramids
17	Ventral median fissure
18	Pyramids
19	Dorsal paraflocculus
20	Pons, transverse fibers
21	Crus cerebri
22	Caudal rhinal sulcus
23	Mamillary bodies
24	Piriform lobe
25	Lateral olfactory tract
26	Lateral olfactory gyrus
27	Medial olfactory tract
28	Olfactory bulb

Figure 1-44   Superficial dissection of the feline head

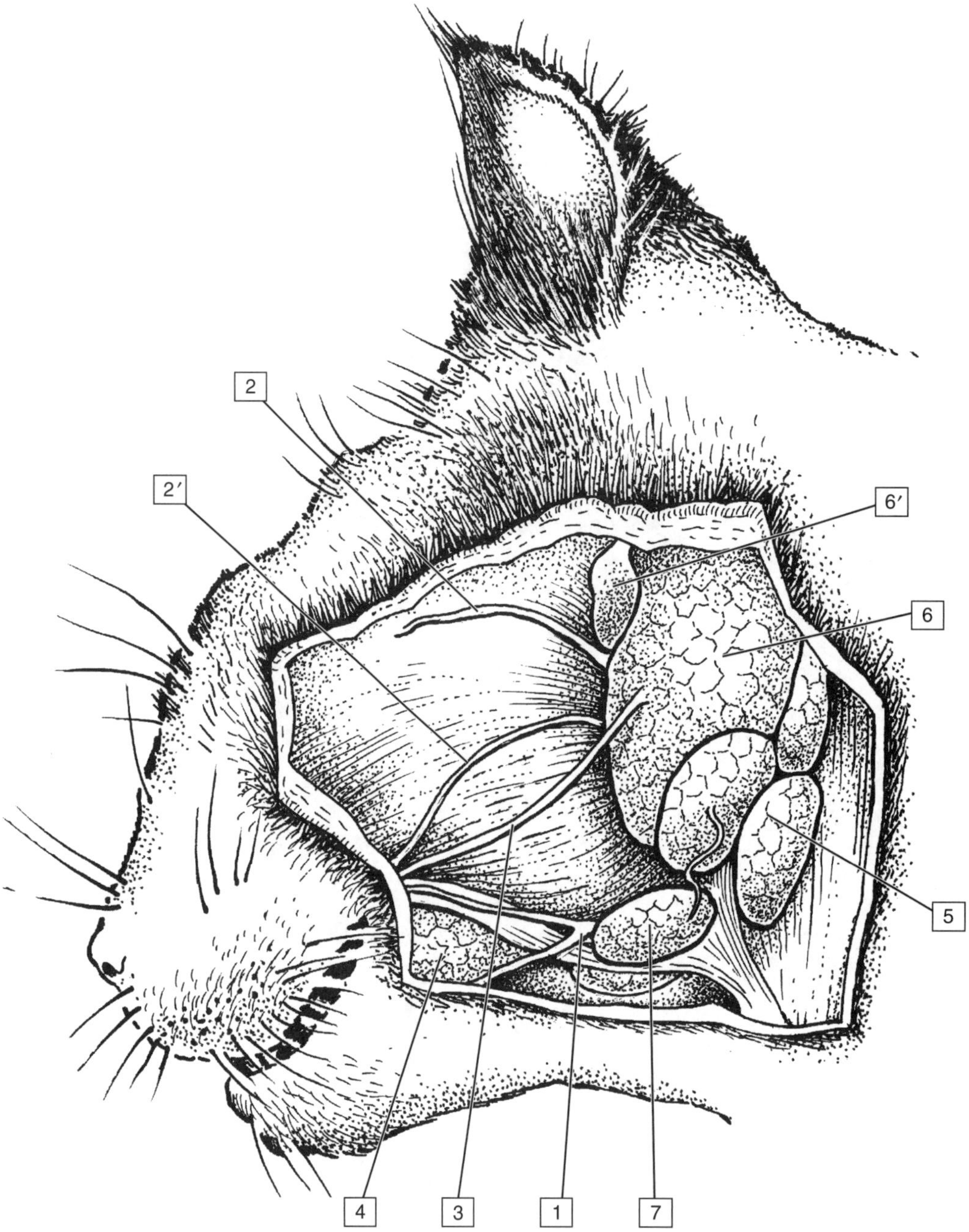

1 Facial vein	5 Mandibular gland
2 Dorsal buccal branch of facial nerve	6 Parotid gland
2′ Ventral buccal branch of facial nerve	6′ Parotid lymph node
3 Parotid duct	7 Mandibular lymph nodes
4 Buccal salivary glands	

Figure 1-45 Deep dissection of the feline head to expose the zygomatic salivary gland

1 Parotid duct, cut

2 Medial pterygoid muscle

3 Parotid gland

4 Mandibular gland

5 Digastricus muscle

6 Mandibular duct

7 Sublingual duct emerging from the rostral end of the monostomatic sublingual salivary gland

8 Zygomatic salivary gland

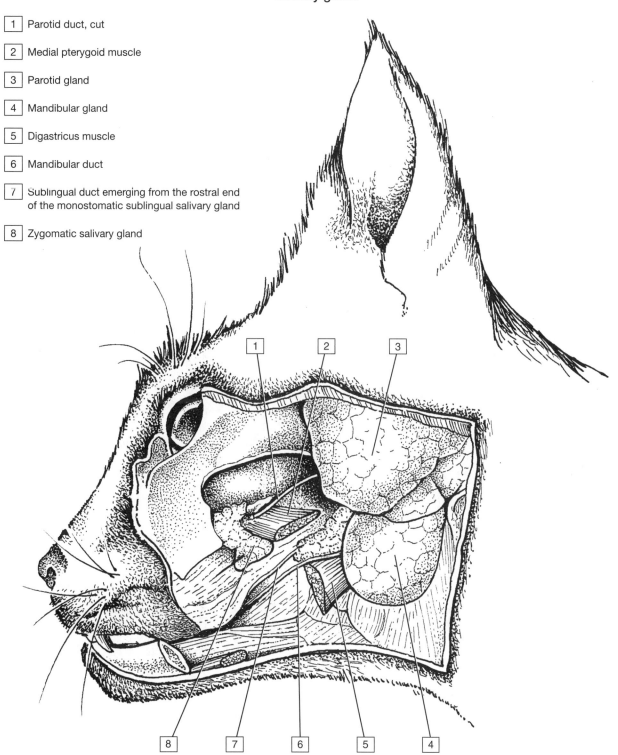

Figure 1-46   *A*, Equine laryngeal skeleton, lateral view, and the intrinsic
muscles of the equine larynx, *B*.

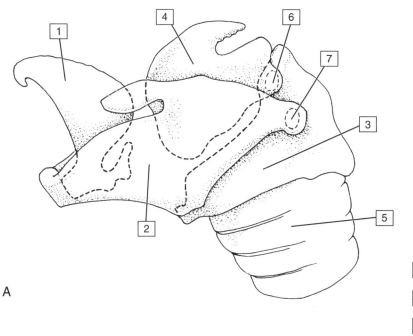

A

1	Epiglottic cartilage
2	Thyroid cartilage
3	Cricoid cartilage
4	Arytenoid cartilage
5	Trachea
6	Cricoarytenoid joint
7	Cricothyroid joint
8	Cricothyroideus
9	Cricoarytenoideus dorsalis
10	Cricoarytenoideus lateralis
11	Vocalis
12	Ventricularis
13	Arytenoideus transversus
14	Laryngeal ventricle

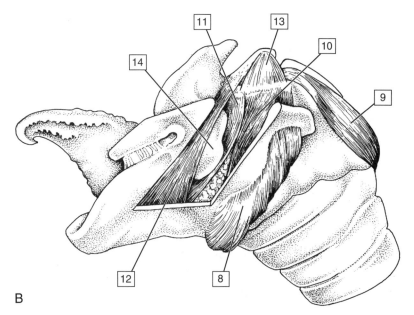

B

Saunders Veterinary Anatomy Coloring Book

Figure 1-47   Transverse section of the equine neck at the level of the fourth
cervical vertebra

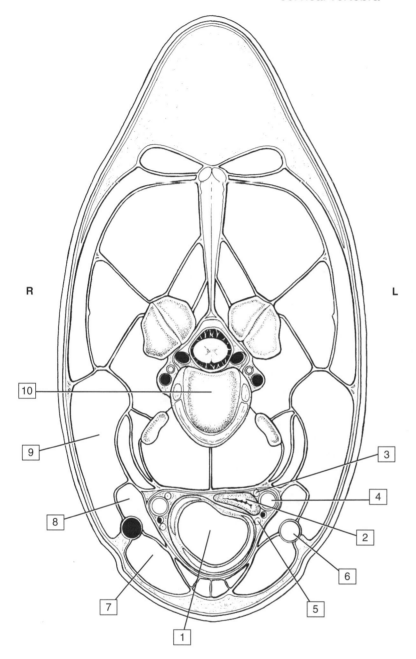

R

L

1 Trachea

2 Esophagus

3 Vagosympathetic trunk

4 Common carotid artery

5 Caudal (recurrent) laryngeal nerve

6 External jugular vein

7 Sternocephalicus

8 Omohyoideus

9 Brachiocephalicus

10 Body of the fourth cervical vertebra

Figure 1-48   Anterior half of the left equine eye, viewed from behind

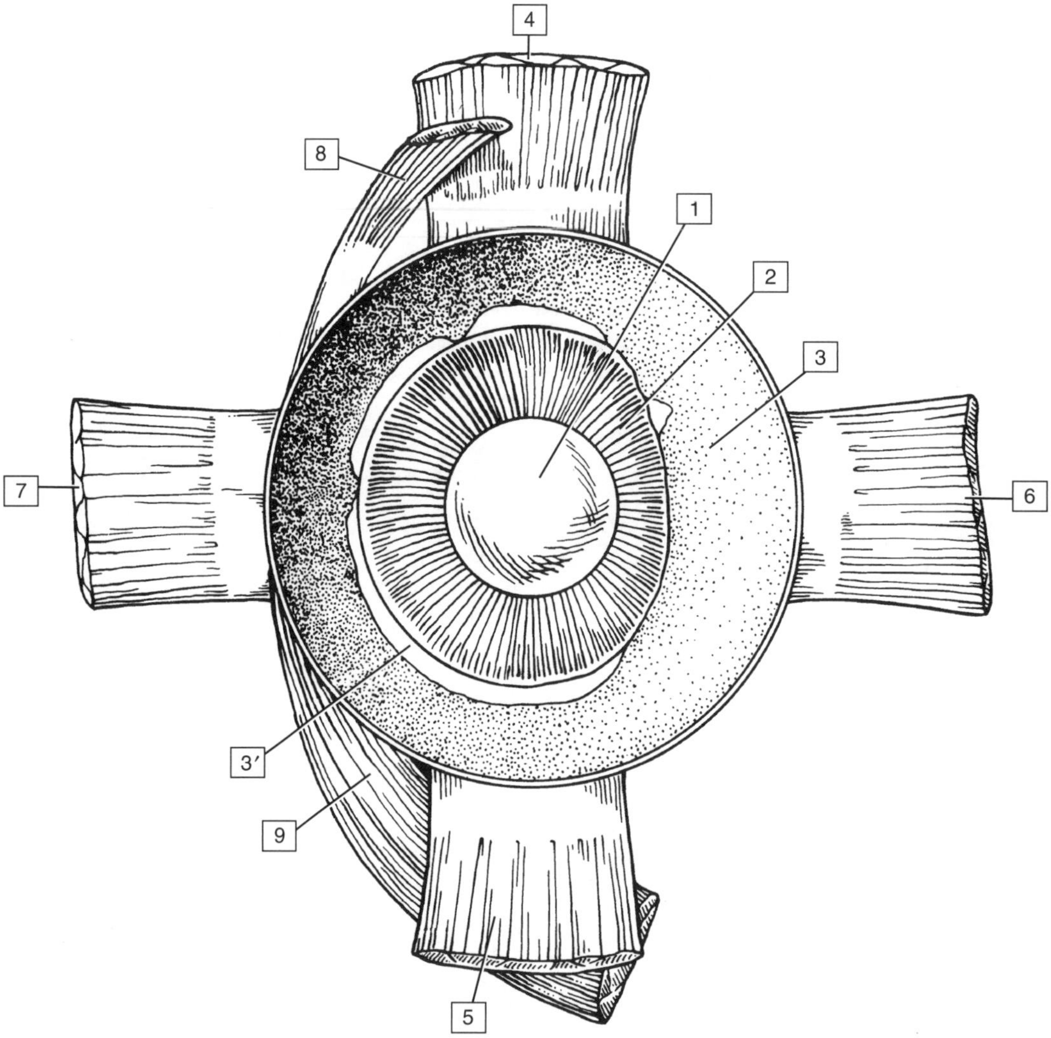

1	Lens
2	Cililary body
3	Choroid covered by pigmented outer layer of retina
3'	Remnants of inner nervous layer of retina, which has been removed
4	Dorsal muscle
5	Ventral muscle
6	Medial muscle
7	Lateral rectus muscle
8	Dorsal oblique muscle
9	Ventral oblique muscle

Figure 1-49   Lateral view of the equine skull

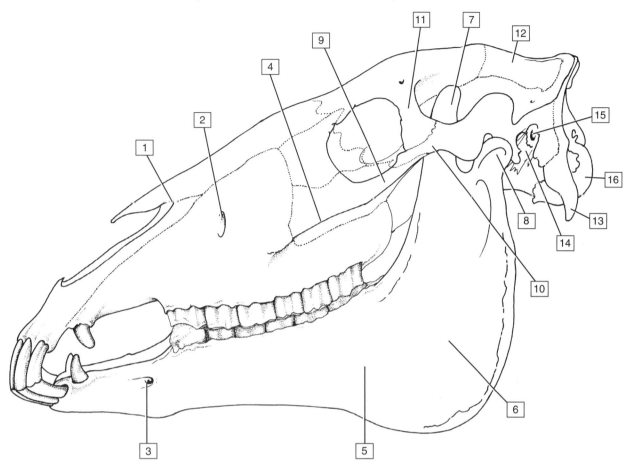

1	Nasoineisive notch	10	Zygomatic process of temporal bone
2	Infraorbital foramen	11	Zygomatic process of frontal bone
3	Mental foramen	12	External sagittal crest
4	Facial crest	13	Paracondylar process
5	Body of mandible	14	Styloid process
6	Ramus of mandible	15	External acoustic meatus
7	Coronoid process	16	Occipital condyle
8	Condylar process		
9	Temporal process of zygomatic bone		

Figure 1-50 Projection of the brain and frontal and maxillary sinuses on the
dorsal surface of the equine skull

The sinuses are filled with casting material. The frontal sinus extends
caudally over the rostral part of the brain and rostrally beyond the level of
the orbit. The circle indicates the center of the brain and the location where a
horse may be shot.

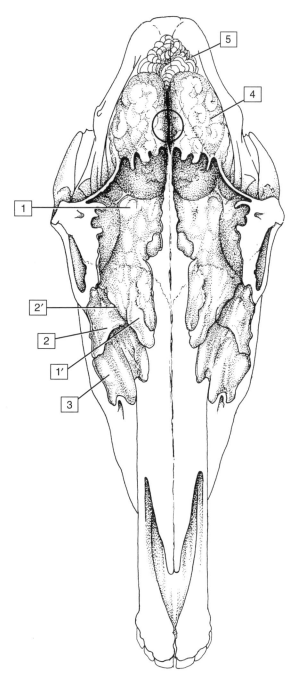

1	Conchofrontal sinus, frontal part	3	Rostral maxillary sinus
1'	Conchofrontal sinus, dorsal conchal part	4	Cerebrum
2	Caudal maxillary sinus	5	Cerebellum
2'	Position of frontomaxillary opening		

Figure 1-51 Structure of a lower equine incisor

A, In situ, sectioned longitudinally; the clinical crown is short in relation to the embedded part of the tooth. *B,* Caudal view; the junction between the clinical crown and the rest of the tooth is not marked. *C,* As a result of wear, the occlusal surface changes; the cup gets smaller and disappears, leaving, for a time, the enamel spot: the dental star appears and changes from a line to a large round spot. *D,* These are sawn sections of a young tooth for comparison. *E,* Longitudinal section of incisor, showing the relationship between the infundibulum and dental cavity; the latter is rostral.

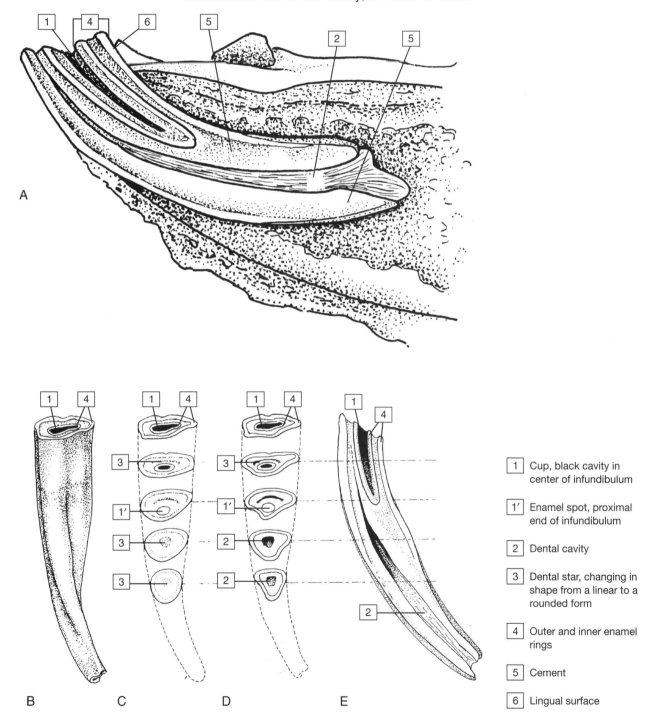

1	Cup, black cavity in center of infundibulum
1'	Enamel spot, proximal end of infundibulum
2	Dental cavity
3	Dental star, changing in shape from a linear to a rounded form
4	Outer and inner enamel rings
5	Cement
6	Lingual surface

Figure 1-52   Equine deep masticatory muscles and right digastricus

A, The deep masticatory muscles of the left side have been exposed by removal
of the left mandibular ramus *(stippled). B,* Medial view of the right digastricus
and some related structures.

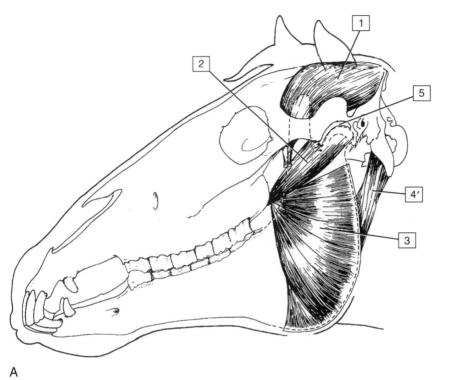

A

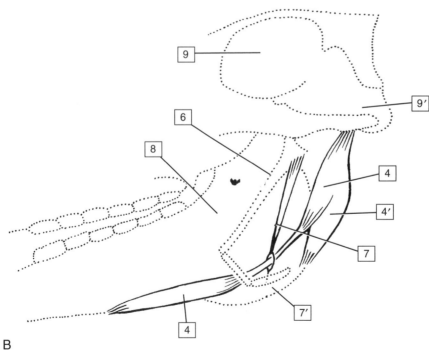

B

1	Temporalis
2	Pterygoideus lateralis
3	Lateral surface of pterygoideus medialis
4	Digastricus
4'	Occipitomandibularis
5	Left temporomandibular joint
6	Stylohyoid
7	Stylohyoideus
7'	Insertion of 7 on thyrohyoid
8	Medial surface of right mandible and mandibular foramen
9	Cranial cavity
9'	Foramen magnum

Figure 1-53   Muscles of the equine pharynx, soft palate, and hyoid apparatus

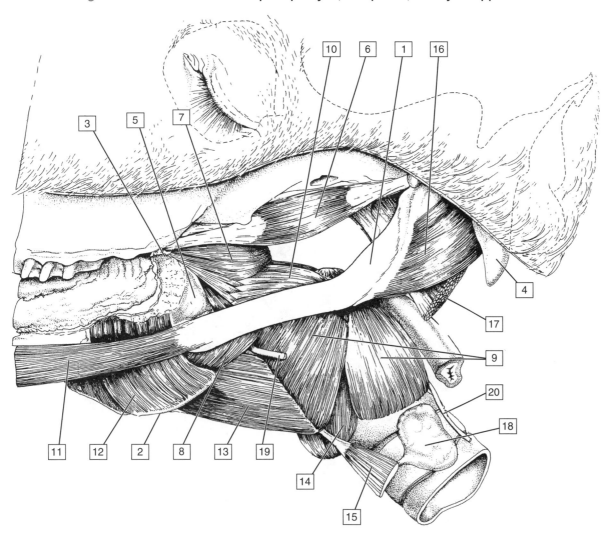

1	Stylohyoid	
2	Thyrohyoid	
3	Hamulus of pterygoid bone	
4	Paracondylar process	
5	Buccopharyngeal fascia	
6	Tensor veli palatini	
7	Rostral pharyngeal constrictor	
8	Middle pharyngeal constrictor	
9	Caudal pharyngeal constrictor (thyro- and cricopharyngeus)	
10	Stylopharyngeus caudalis	

11	Styloglossus
12	Hyoglossus
13	Thyrohyoideus
14	Cricothyroideus
15	Sternothyroideus
16	Occipitohyoideus
17	Longus capitis (stump)
18	Thyroid gland
19	Cranial laryngeal nerve
20	Caudal (recurrent) laryngeal nerve

Figure 1-54   Dissection of the equine orbit

The zygomatic arch and periorbita have been removed.

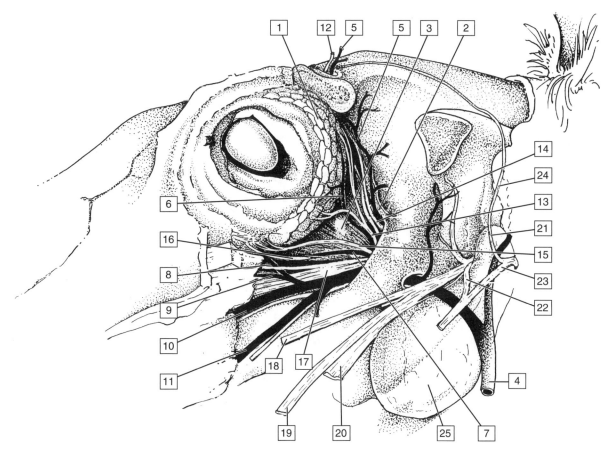

1	Lacrimal gland	14	Trochlear n.
2	Periorbita	15	Zygomatic n.
3	Lateral rectus	16	Oculomotor n.
4	Maxillary a.	17	Rostral branches of maxillary n.
5	Supraorbital a.		
6	Lacrimal a.	18	Buccal n.
7	Muscular branch of external ophthalmic a.	19	Lingual n.
		20	Inferior alveolar n.
8	Malar a.	21	Masticatory n.
9	Infraorbital a.	22	Auriculotemporal n.
10	Major palatine a.	23	Facial n.
11	Buccal a.	24	Auriculopalpebral n.
12	Supraorbital n.	25	Guttural pouch
13	Lacrimal n.		

Figure 1-55   Transection of the equine neck at the level of the fourth cervical vertebra

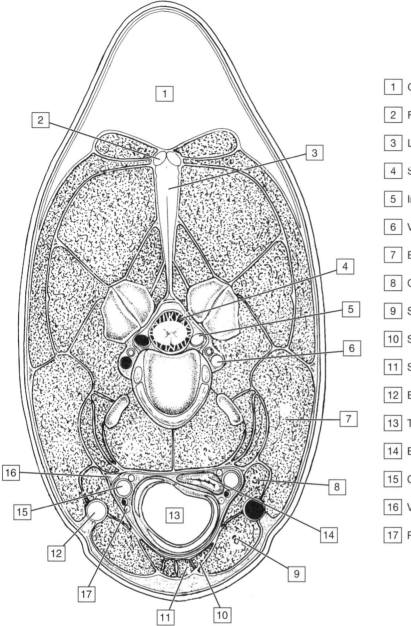

1   Crest

2   Funicular part of nuchal ligament

3   Laminar part of nuchal ligament

4   Subarachnoid space

5   Internal vertebral venous plexus

6   Vertebral artery and vein

7   Brachiocephalicus

8   Omohyoideus

9   Sternocephalicus

10   Sternothyroideus

11   Sternohyoideus

12   External jugular vein

13   Trachea

14   Esophagus

15   Common carotid artery

16   Vagosympathetic trunk

17   Recurrent laryngeal nerve

Figure 1-56   Principal arteries of the equine head

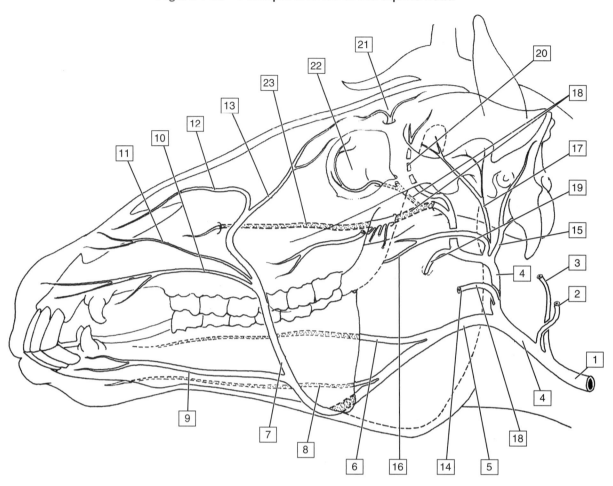

1	Common carotid a.	13	Angularis oculi a.
2	Occipital a.	14	Masseteric a.
3	Internal carotid a.	15	Caudal auricular a.
4	External carotid a.	16	Transverse facial a., displaced ventrally for clarity
5	Linguofacial a.	17	Superficial temporal a.
6	Lingual a.	18	Maxillary a.
7	Facial a.	19	Inferior alveolar a.
8	Sublingual a.	20	Caudal deep temporal a.
9	Inferior labial a.	21	Supraorbital a.
10	Superior labial a.	22	Malar a.
11	Lateral nasal a.	23	Infraorbital a.
12	Dorsal nasal a.		

Figure 1-57   Bovine skull with mandible

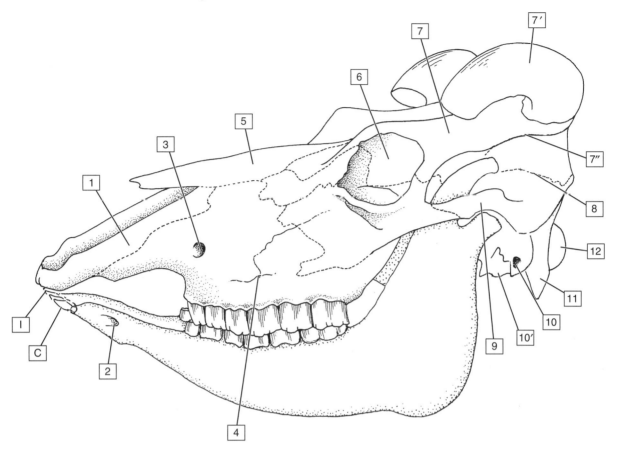

1	Incisive bone	7″	Temporal line
2	Mental foramen	8	Temporal fossa
3	Infraorbital foramen	9	Zygomatic arch
4	Facial tuberosity	10	External acoustic meatus
5	Nasal bone	10′	Tympanic bulla
6	Orbit	11	Paracondylar process
7	Frontal bone	12	Occipital condyle
7′	Horn surrounding cornual process of frontal bone	I	Incisors
		C	Canine tooth

Figure 1-58 Transverse section of the bovine neck

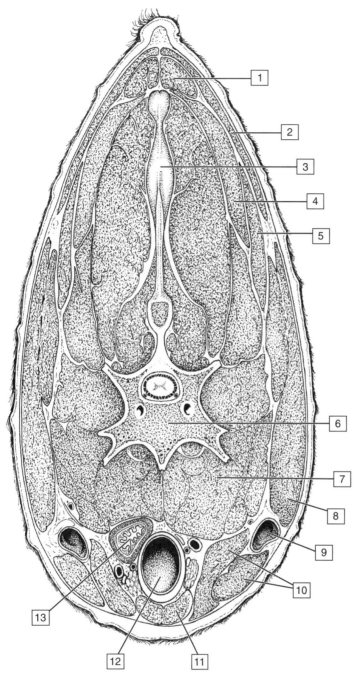

1 Rhomboideus

2 Trapezius

3 Nuchal ligament

4 Splenius

5 Omotransversarius

6 Vertebra

7 Longus colli

8 Brachiocephalicus

9 External jugular vein in jugular groove

10 Sternocephalicus, mandibular, and mastoid parts

11 Combined sternohyoideus and sternothyroideus

12 Trachea

13 Esophagus (ventral to it, nerves, blood vessels, and thymus)

Figure 1-59   Lateral view of the connection of the pharynx with the base
of the bovine skull

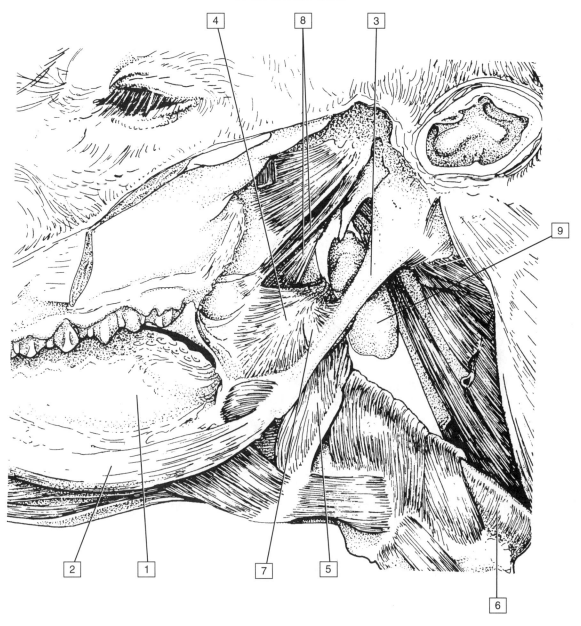

1	Root of tongue	6	Esophagus
2	Styloglossus	7	Pharyngeal dilator (stylopharyngeus caudalis)
3	Stylohyoid	8	Tensor and levator veli palatini
4	Rostral pharyngeal constrictor	9	Medial retropharyngeal lymph node
5	Middle pharyngeal constrictor		

Figure 1-60 Right bovine eye cut along orbital axis, rostromedial surface

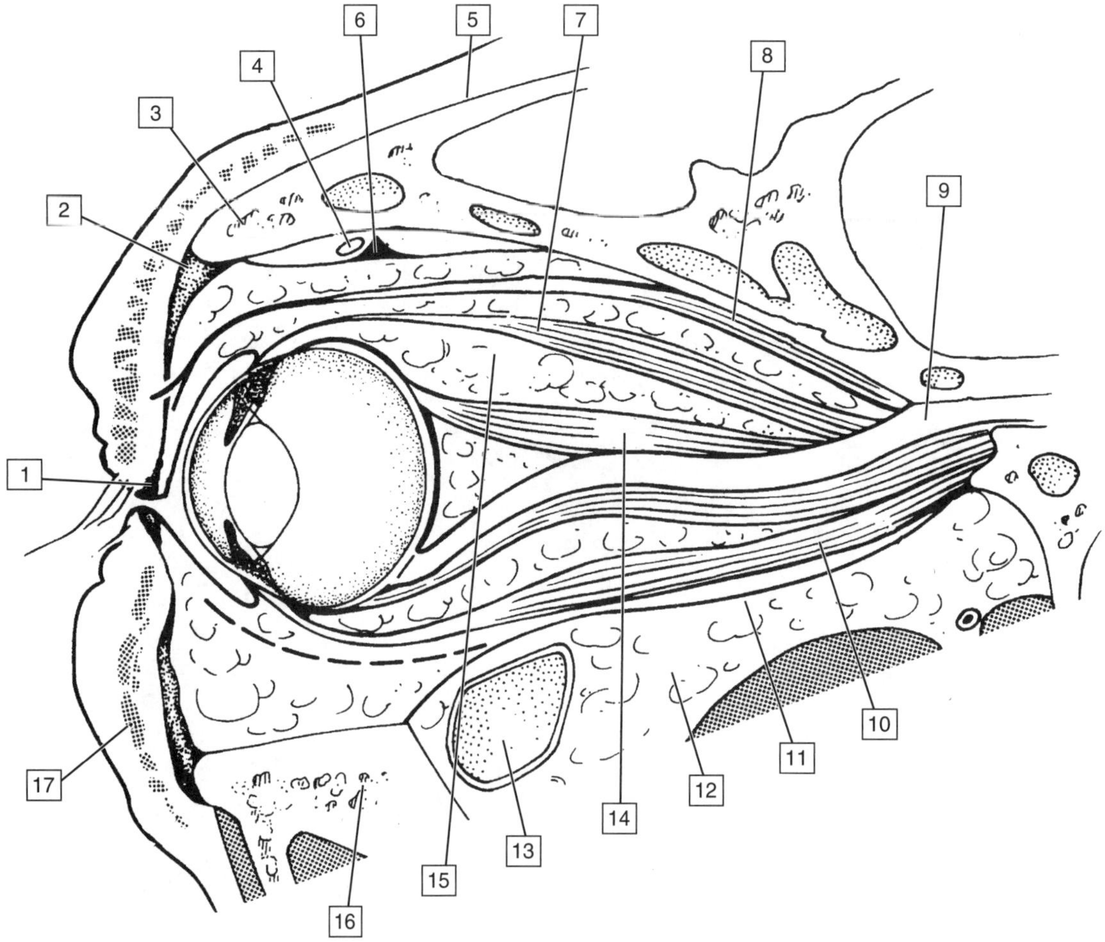

1	Tarsus	10	Ventral rectus muscle
2	Orbital septum	11	Periorbita
3	Orbital margin	12	Extraorbital fat
4	Dorsal oblique muscle	13	Lacrimal bulla, a caudal recess of the maxillary sinus
5	Periosteum of face	14	Retractor bulbi
6	Trochlea	15	Intraperiorbital fat
7	Dorsal rectus muscle	16	Zygomatic arch
8	Levator palpebrae superioris	17	Orbicularis
9	Optic nerve in optic foramen		

Figure 1-61   Connections of the pharynx and larynx with the base of the bovine skull and the tongue

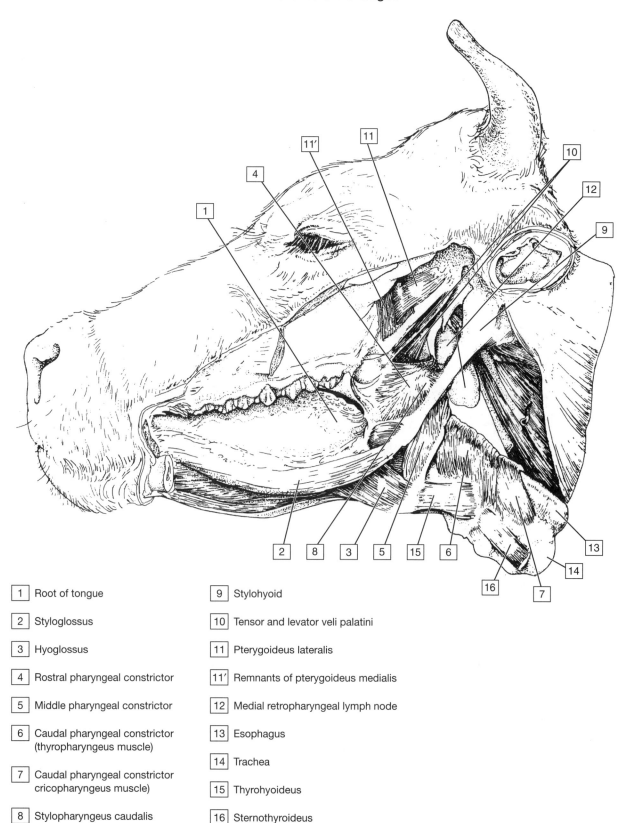

1 Root of tongue	9 Stylohyoid
2 Styloglossus	10 Tensor and levator veli palatini
3 Hyoglossus	11 Pterygoideus lateralis
4 Rostral pharyngeal constrictor	11′ Remnants of pterygoideus medialis
5 Middle pharyngeal constrictor	12 Medial retropharyngeal lymph node
6 Caudal pharyngeal constrictor (thyropharyngeus muscle)	13 Esophagus
7 Caudal pharyngeal constrictor cricopharyngeus muscle)	14 Trachea
8 Stylopharyngeus caudalis	15 Thyrohyoideus
	16 Sternothyroideus

Figure 1-62   Branching of the bovine left common carotid artery

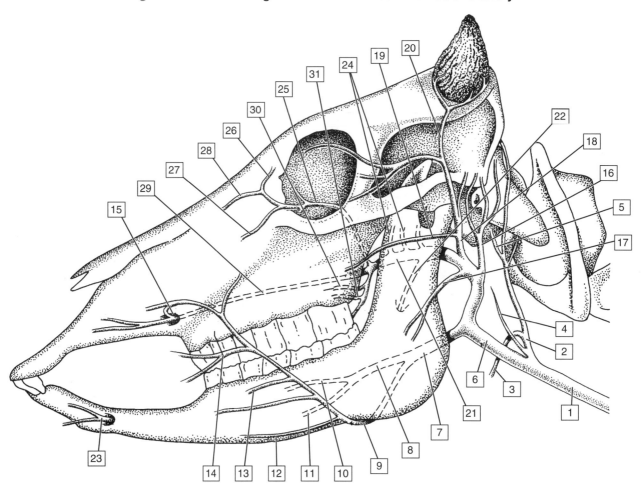

1 Common carotid a.	12 Submental a.	23 Mental a.
2 Occipital a.	13 Inferior labial a.	24 Rostral and caudal branches to rete mirabile
3 Ascending palatine a.	14 Superior labial a.	
4 Remnant of internal carotid a.	15 Infraorbital foramen	25 Malar a.
5 Medial meningeal a.	16 Caudal auricular a.	26 Angular a. of the eye
6 External carotid a.	17 Masseteric branch	27 Caudal lateral nasal a.
7 Linguofacial trunk	18 Superficial temporal a.	28 Dorsal nasal a.
8 Lingual a.	19 Transverse facial a.	29 Infraorbital a.
9 Facial a.	20 Cornual a.	30 Sphenopalatine a.
10 Deep lingual a.	21 Maxillary a.	31 Major and minor palatine a.
11 Sublingual a.	22 Inferior alveolar a.	

Saunders Veterinary Anatomy Coloring Book
Copyright © 2011 by Saunders, an imprint of Elsevier Inc.

Figure 1-63   Lateral view of the skull of a sheep

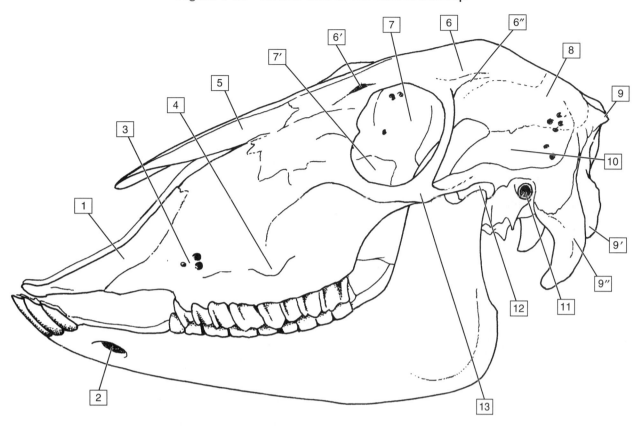

1	Incisive bone	7'	Lacrimal bulla
2	Mental foramen	8	Parietal bone
3	Infraorbital foramina	9	External occipital protuberance
4	Facial tuberosity		
5	Nasal bone	9'	Occipital condyle
6	Frontal bone	9"	Paracondylar process
6'	Supraorbital foramen and groove	10	Temporal fossa
		11	External acoustic meatus
6"	Temporal line	12	Temporomandibular joint
7	Orbit	13	Zygomatic arch

Figure 1-64   Porcine head, superficial dissection

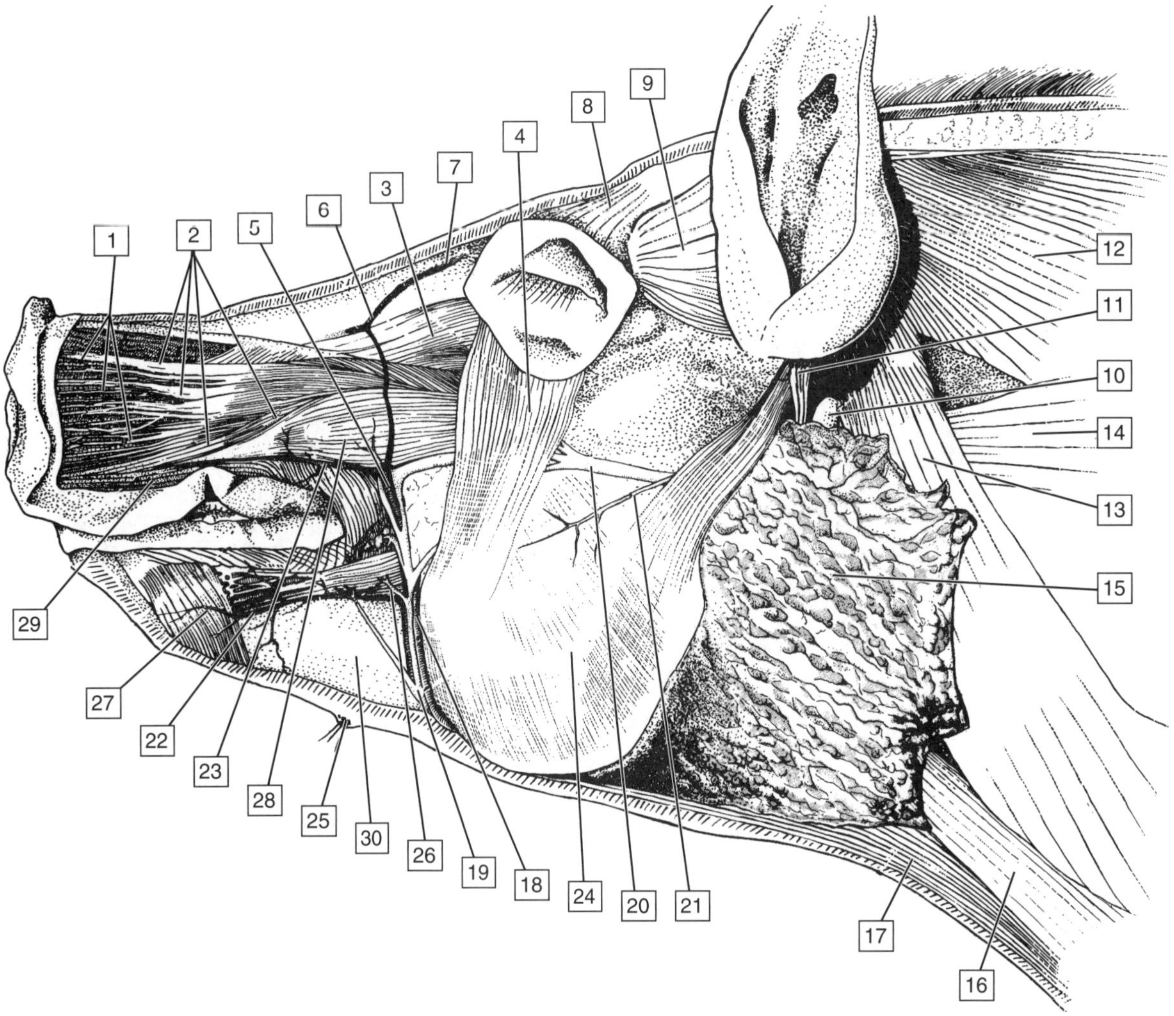

1 Cut fasciculi of levator nasolabialis	12 Trapezius	21 Transverse facial nerve
2 Caninus	13 Cleido-occipitalis	22 Inferior labial vein
3 Levator labii superioris	14 Omotransversarius	23 Superior labial vein
4 Malaris	15 Parotid gland	24 Masseter
5 Facial vein	16 Sternocephalicus	25 Mental hairs and gland
6 Dorsal nasal vein	17 Sternohyoideus	26 Depressor labii inferioris
7 Frontal vein	18 Parotid duct	27 Mentalis
8 Levator anguli oculi	19 Ventral and dorsal buccal branches of facial nerve	28 Depressor labii superioris
9 Frontoscutularis	20 Ventral and dorsal buccal branches of facial nerve	29 Orbicularis oris
10 Lateral retropharyneal lymph node		30 Mandible
11 Parotidoauricularis		

Figure 1-65   Paramedian section of the porcine skull

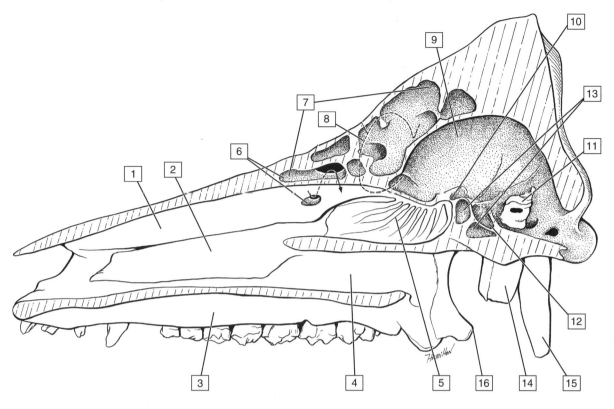

1 Dorsal turbinate bone, fenestrated at 6 to show conchal sinus	**9** Cranial cavity
2 Ventral turbinate bone	**10** Optic canal
3 Hard palate	**11** Petrous temporal bone
4 Choana	**12** Fossa for hypophysis
5 Ethmoturbinates in fundus of nasal cavity	**13** Sphenoid sinus
6 Conchal sinus	**14** Tympanic bulla
7 Portion of frontal sinus exposed by paramedian saw cut	**15** Paracondylar process
8 Position of orbit	**16** Hamulus of pterygoid bone

Figure 1-66   Median section of the head of a 4-week-old pig

The nasal septum has been removed.

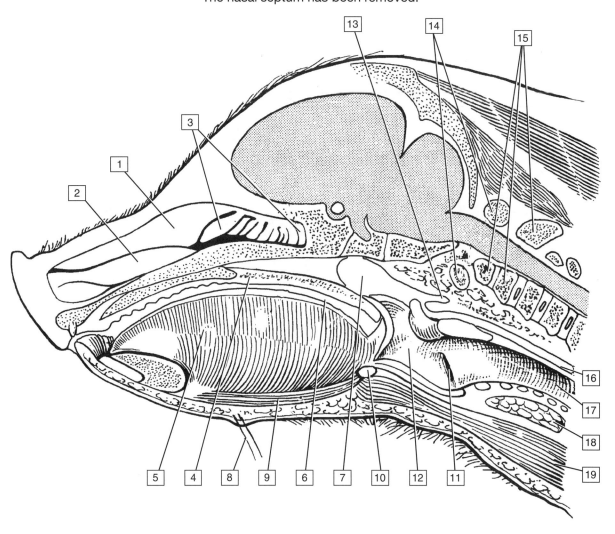

1 Dorsal nasal concha	11 Laryngeal ventricle
2 Ventral nasal concha	12 Larynx
3 Ethmoidal conchae	13 Pharyngeal diverticulum
4 Soft palate	14 Atlas
5 Tongue	15 Axis
6 Oropharynx	16 Esophagus
7 Nasopharynx	17 Trachea
8 Mental hairs	18 Thyroid gland
9 Geniohyoideus	19 Sternohyoideus
10 Basihyoid	

Figure 1-67   Transverse section of the ventral neck of swine

A, Transverse section of the ventral neck slightly cranial to the manubrium sterni.
B, The area within the broken line represents the topography at the slightly
more caudal level of the first ribs. *C*, Pig held on its back for cranial vena cava
venipuncture; see needle in position.

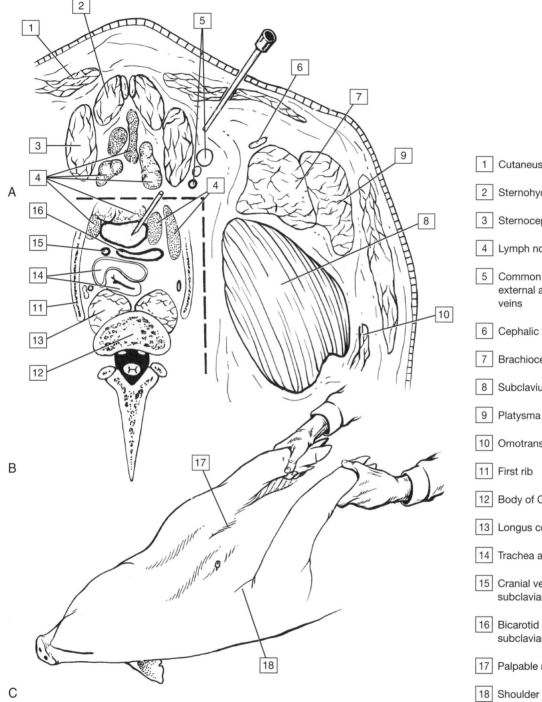

1	Cutaneus colli
2	Sternohyoideus
3	Sternocephalicus
4	Lymph nodes and thymus
5	Common carotid artery and external and internal jugular veins
6	Cephalic vein
7	Brachiocephalicus
8	Subclavius
9	Platysma
10	Omotransversarius
11	First rib
12	Body of C7
13	Longus colli
14	Trachea and esophagus
15	Cranial vena cava and left subclavian artery
16	Bicarotid trunk and right subclavian artery
17	Palpable manubrium sterni
18	Shoulder joint

Figure 1-68 The lymph centers of the swine head and neck

The arrows indicate lymph flow.

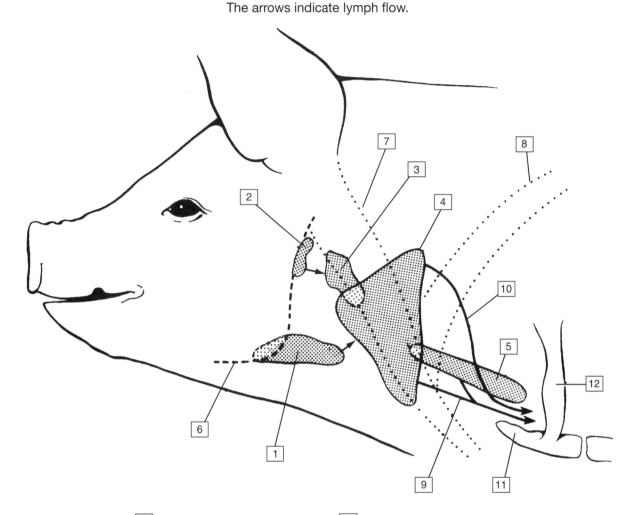

1 Mandibular lymph center	8 Subclavius
2 Parotid lymph center	9 Tracheal lymph trunk
3 Retropharyngeal lymph center	10 Lymph from dorsal superficial cervical nodes
4 Superficial cervical lymph center	
5 Deep cervical lymph center	11 Manubrium sterni
6 Mandible	12 First rib
7 Brachiocephalicus	

Saunders Veterinary Anatomy Coloring Book
Copyright © 2011 by Saunders, an imprint of Elsevier Inc.

Figure 1-69   Avian skull

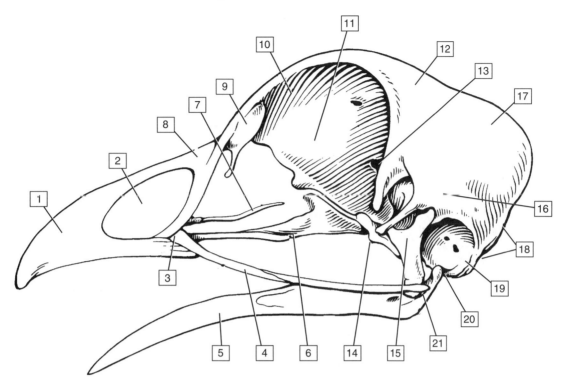

1 Premaxilla	12 Frontal bone
2 Nasal aperture	13 Optic foramen
3 Maxilla	14 Pterygoid bone
4 Jugal arch	15 Quadrate bone
5 Mandible	16 Temporal bone
6 Palatine bone	17 Parietal bone
7 Vomer	18 Occipital bone
8 Nasal bone	19 Tympanic cavity with cochlear and vestibular windows
9 Lacrimal bone	20 Splenoid bone
10 Orbit	21 Articular bone
11 Interoribital septum	

Figure 1-70   Ventral view of the dissected avian neck

The inset shows a transverse section through the middle of the neck.

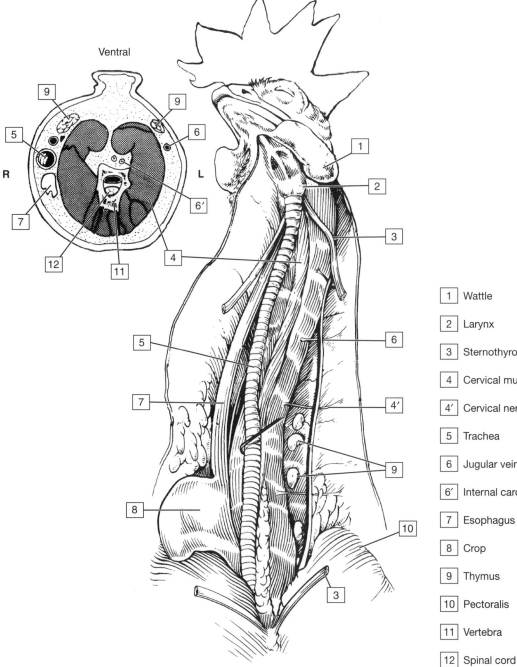

1	Wattle
2	Larynx
3	Sternothyroideus, cut
4	Cervical muscles
4′	Cervical nerve
5	Trachea
6	Jugular vein and vagus
6′	Internal carotid arteries
7	Esophagus
8	Crop
9	Thymus
10	Pectoralis
11	Vertebra
12	Spinal cord

Figure 1-71 Dorsal view of the (*A*) canine, (*B*) feline, (*C*) porcine, (*D*) bovine, and (*E*) equine tongue and epiglottis

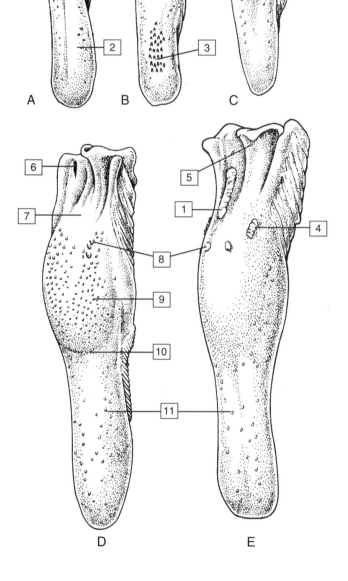

1 Palatine tonsil	7 Root of tongue
2 Median groove	8 Vallate papillae
3 Filiform papillae	9 Torus linguae
4 Foliate papillae	10 Fossa linguae
5 Epiglottis	11 Fungiform papillae
6 Tonsillar sinus	

Figure 1-72   Canine, porcine, bovine, and equine major salivary glands

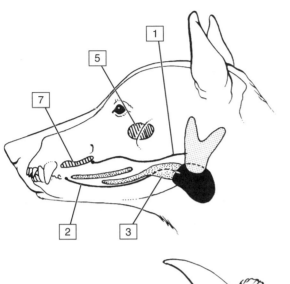
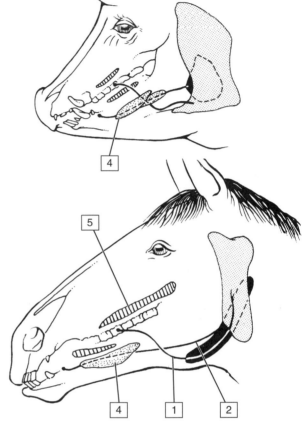
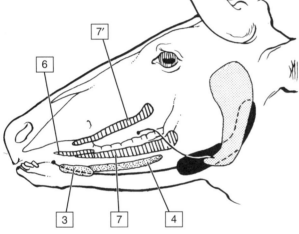

1	Parotid duct		5	Dorsal buccal glands (zygomatic gland in the dog)
2	Mandibular duct		6	Middle buccal glands
3	Compact (monostomatic) part of sublingual gland		7	Ventral buccal glands
4	Diffuse (polystomatic) part of sublingual gland		7'	Dorsal buccal gland

Figure 1-73   Median sections of the (*A*) equine, (*B*) bovine, (*C*) porcine, and
(*D*) canine hypophysis

The rostral extremity of the gland is to the left.

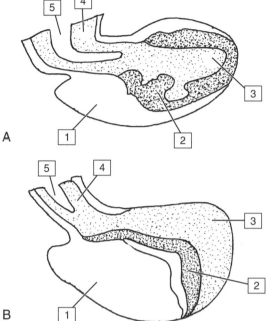

A

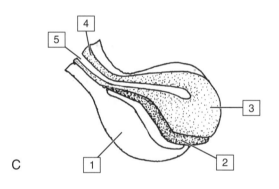

B

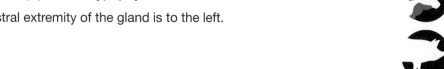

C

D

1	Adenohypophysis
2	Intermediate part
3	Neurohypophysis
4	Hypophysial stalk
5	Recess of third ventricle

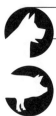

Figure 1-74   Canine and porcine third eyelid

A, Left eye of dog showing third eyelid and lacrimal apparatus. *B,* Isolated cartilage of the third eyelid and associated glands of a pig.

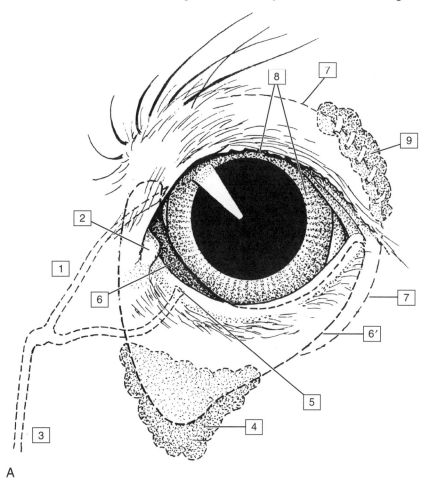

A

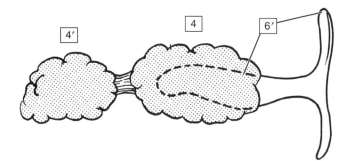

B

1	Upper canaliculus
2	Lacrimal caruncle
3	Nasolacrimal duct
4	Gland of third eyelid
4′	Deep gland of third eyelid
5	Punctum lacrimale
6	Third eyelid
6′	Cartilage of third eyelid
7	Position of conjunctival fornix
8	Pupil
9	Lacrimal gland

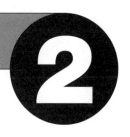

Figure 2-1   Transection of the canine vertebral column to show the formation
of a spinal nerve

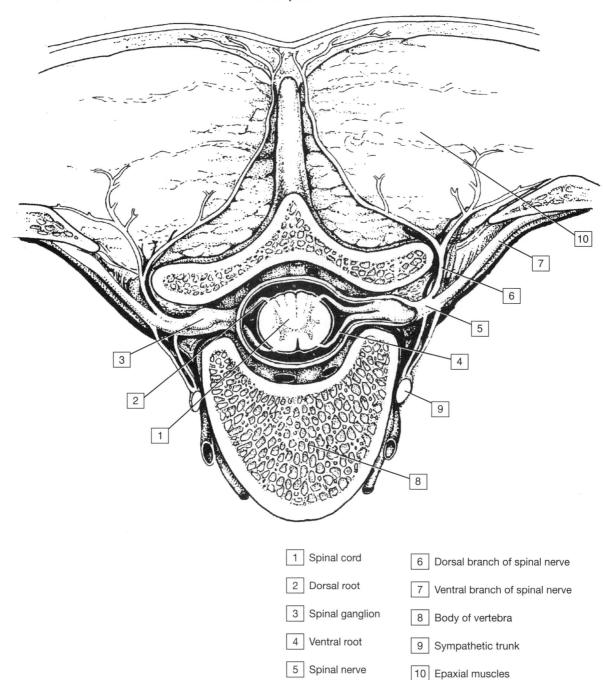

1	Spinal cord	6	Dorsal branch of spinal nerve
2	Dorsal root	7	Ventral branch of spinal nerve
3	Spinal ganglion	8	Body of vertebra
4	Ventral root	9	Sympathetic trunk
5	Spinal nerve	10	Epaxial muscles

Figure 2-2 Cervical and thoracic vertebrae of the dog

A, Axis, lateral view. *B,* Fifth vertebra, lateral view. *C,* Thoracic vertebra, left lateral view

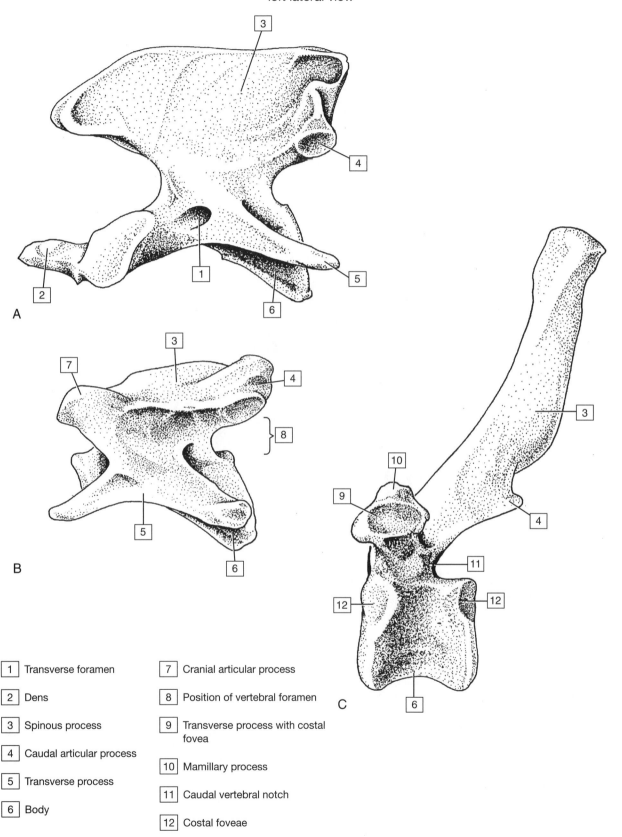

1 Transverse foramen	7	Cranial articular process
2 Dens	8	Position of vertebral foramen
3 Spinous process	9	Transverse process with costal fovea
4 Caudal articular process	10	Mamillary process
5 Transverse process	11	Caudal vertebral notch
6 Body	12	Costal foveae

Figure 2-3 Ventral muscles of the canine neck and thorax

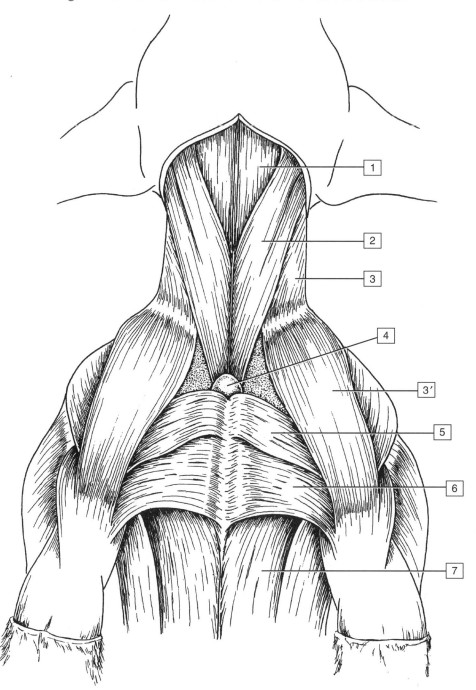

1	Combined sternohyoideus and sternothyroideus	4	Manubrium of sternum
2	Sternocephalicus	5	Pectoralis descendens
3	Brachiocephalicus: cleidocervicalis	6	Pectoralis transversus
3'	Brachiocephalicus: cleidocervicalis	7	Pectoralis profundus

Figure 2-4   Transverse section of the canine back at the level of the first lumbar vertebra

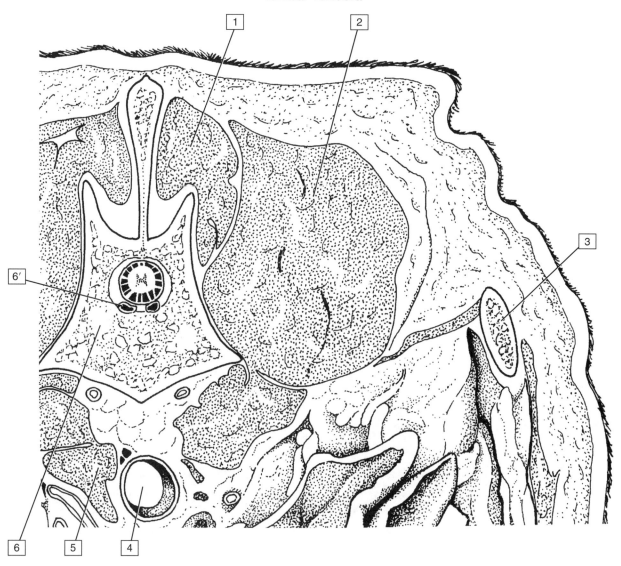

1	Multifidus and spinalis	5	Right crus of diaphragm
2	Longissimus and iliocostalis	6	First lumbar vertebra
3	Last rib	6′	Internal vertebral venous plexus
4	Aorta		

Figure 2-5   Muscles associated with the canine atlanto-occipital and atlantoaxial joints, lateral view

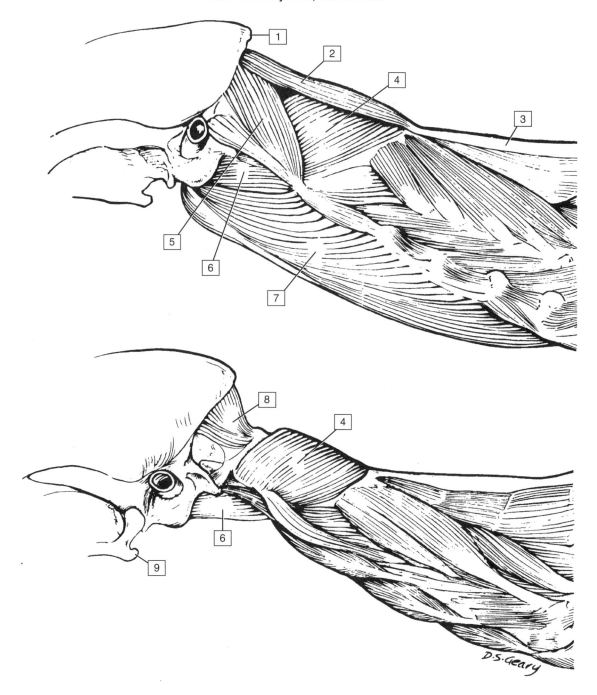

1	External occipital protuberance	6	Rectus capitis ventralis
2	Rectus capitis dorsalis major	7	Longus capitis
3	Nuchal ligament	8	Rectus capitis dorsalis minor
4	Obliquus capitis caudalis	9	Angular process of mandible
5	Obliquus capitis cranialis		

Figure 2-6   Peripheral distribution of canine sympathetic and parasympathetic divisions

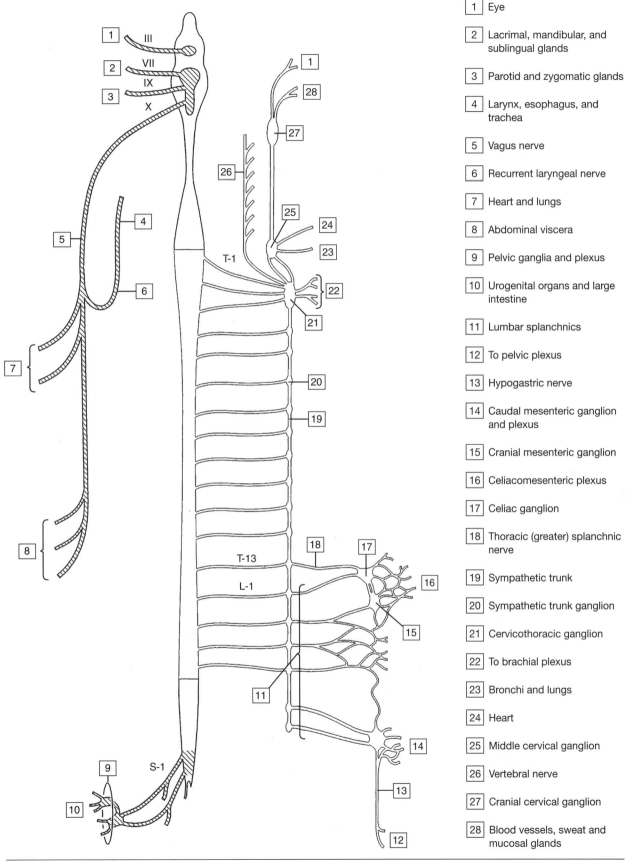

1   Eye

2   Lacrimal, mandibular, and sublingual glands

3   Parotid and zygomatic glands

4   Larynx, esophagus, and trachea

5   Vagus nerve

6   Recurrent laryngeal nerve

7   Heart and lungs

8   Abdominal viscera

9   Pelvic ganglia and plexus

10   Urogenital organs and large intestine

11   Lumbar splanchnics

12   To pelvic plexus

13   Hypogastric nerve

14   Caudal mesenteric ganglion and plexus

15   Cranial mesenteric ganglion

16   Celiacomesenteric plexus

17   Celiac ganglion

18   Thoracic (greater) splanchnic nerve

19   Sympathetic trunk

20   Sympathetic trunk ganglion

21   Cervicothoracic ganglion

22   To brachial plexus

23   Bronchi and lungs

24   Heart

25   Middle cervical ganglion

26   Vertebral nerve

27   Cranial cervical ganglion

28   Blood vessels, sweat and mucosal glands

Figure 2-7   Canine epaxial muscles

Each of the named muscles shown can be present, spanning other vertebrae, thus overlapping and obscuring their individual nature.

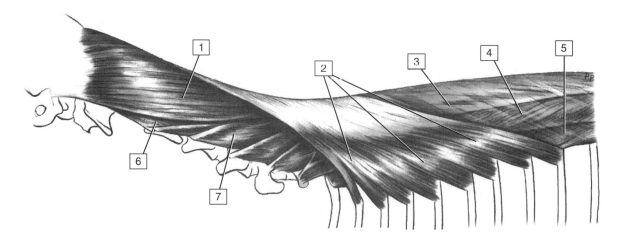

1	Splenius	5	Iliocostalis
2	Serratus dorsalis cranialis	6	Longissimus capitis
3	Spinalis at semispinalis	7	Longissimus cervicis
4	Longissimus		

Figure 2-8　Equine sternum and costal cartilages, lateral view

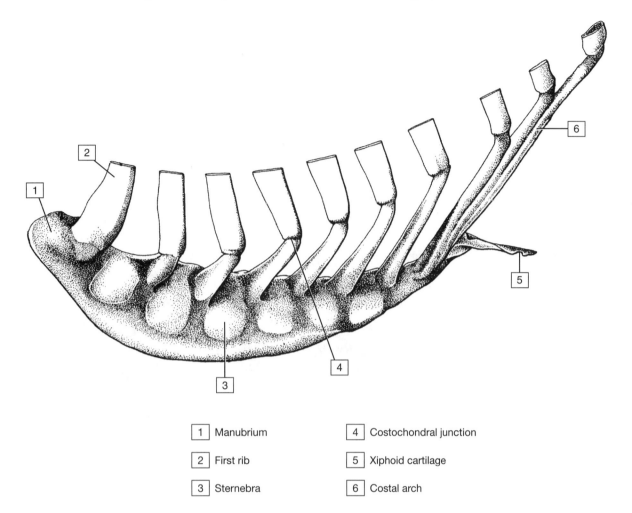

1	Manubrium	4	Costochondral junction
2	First rib	5	Xiphoid cartilage
3	Sternebra	6	Costal arch

Figure 2-9   Superficial dissection of the equine head

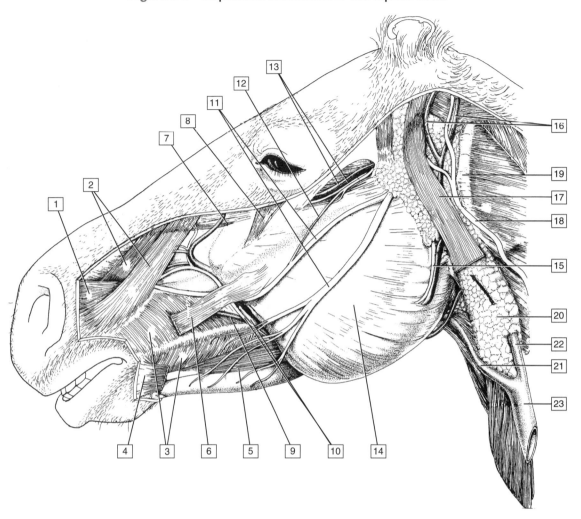

1 Caninus

2 Levator nasolabialis

3 Buccinator

4 Stump of cutaneous muscle joining orbicularis oris

5 Depressor labii inferioris

6 Zygomaticus

7 Levator labii superioris

8 Malaris

9 Parotid duct

10 Facial artery and vein

11 Buccal branches of facial nerve

12 Rostral communicating branch of auriculotemporal nerve

13 Transverse facial artery and vein and transverse facial branch of auriculotemporal nerve

14 Masseter

15 Masseteric artery and vein

16 Auricular veins

17 Parotidauricularis

18 Great auricular nerve (C2)

19 Wing of atlas

20 Parotid gland

21 Linguofacial vein

22 Maxillary vein

23 External jugular vein

Figure 2-10   Segmentation of the bovine paraxial mesoderm

10-mm bovine embryo (*top*) together with two stages in the development of the vertebrae and related vessels and nerves. The arrows show the formation of each vertebra from two pairs of adjacent somites.

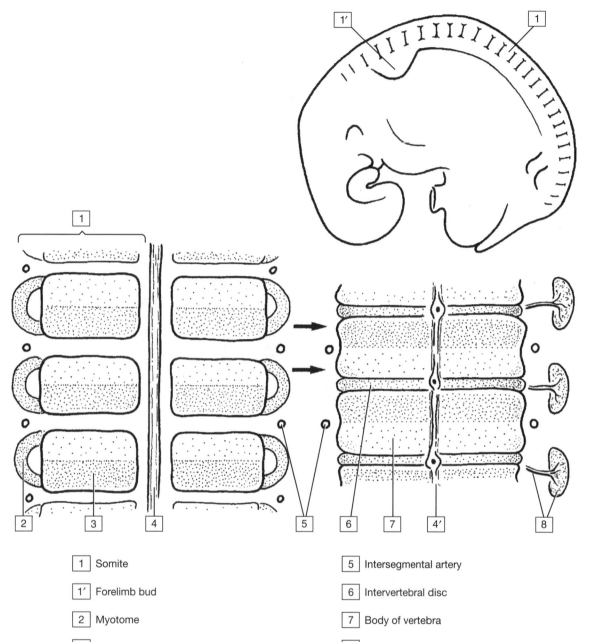

1	Somite	5	Intersegmental artery
1′	Forelimb bud	6	Intervertebral disc
2	Myotome	7	Body of vertebra
3	Sclerotome	8	Myotome with segmental nerve
4	Notochord		
4′	Notochord giving rise to the nucleus pulposus in the center of the intervertebral disc (6)		

Figure 2-11   Bovine lumbar intervertebral disc

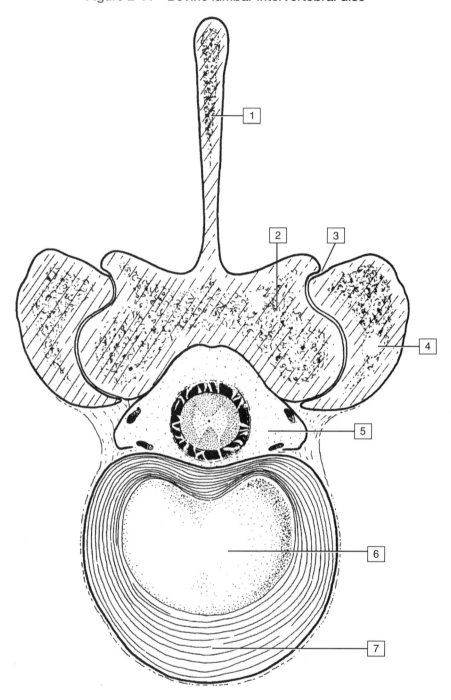

1 Spinous process

2 Lamina

3 Synovial intervertebral joint

4 Articular process of adjacent vertebra

5 Vertebral canal with contents (spinal cord and meninges surrounded by epidural fat)

6 Nucleus pulposus

7 Anulus fibrosus

Figure 2-12 Caudal part of the bovine vertebral canal and its contents

Epidural injection sites are indicated by the needles.

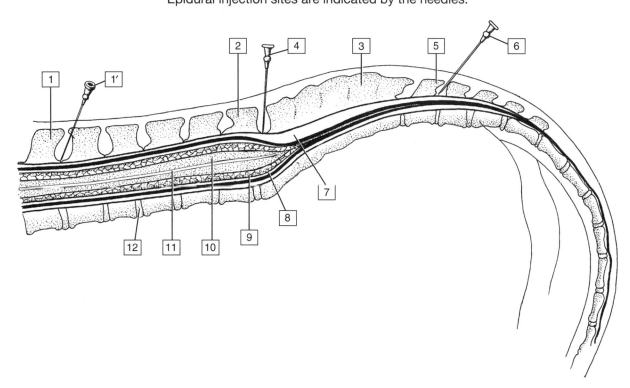

1	First lumbar vertebra	
1′	Needle in position for flank anesthesia	
2	Last lumbar vertebra (L6)	
3	Sacrum	
4	Needle in lumbosacral space	
5	First caudal vertebra	
6	Needle between first and second caudal vertebrae (tail block)	

7	Epidural space
8	Dura mater
9	Subarachnoid space
10	Spinal cord
11	Central canal
12	Intervertebral disc

Figure 2-13   The connections of the major veins with the bovine vertebral plexus-azygous system

Note, specifically, the connections between the internal vertebral plexus and the intercostal veins and between the plexus and the branches of the vertebral vein.

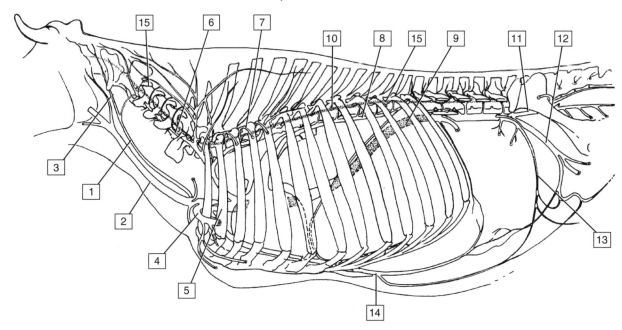

1 Internal jugular v.	10 Intercostal v.
2 External jugular v.	11 Internal iliac v.
3 Occipital v.	12 External iliac v.
4 Axillary v.	13 Deep circumflex iliac v.
5 Cranial vena cava	14 Cranial epigastric v.
6 Vertebral v.	15 Internal vertebral plexus, stippled in the vertebral canal
7 Supreme intercostal v.	
8 Left azygous v.	
9 Caudal vena cava	

Figure 2-14   Avian uropygial (preen) gland, dorsal view

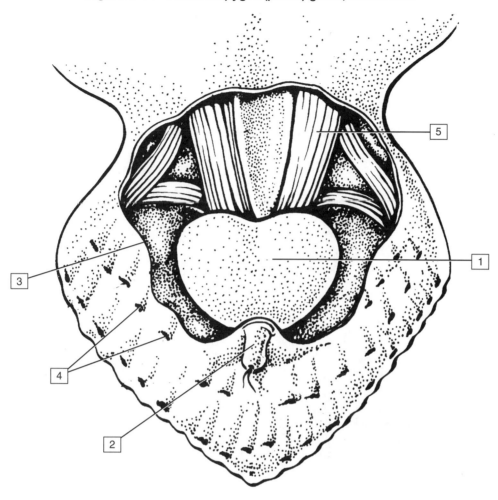

1	Uropygial gland	4	Feather follicles
2	Papilla of uropygial gland through which the secretion is extruded	5	Caudal vertebrae and associated muscles
3	Cut edge of skin		

Figure 2-15   The canine (*A*), equine (*B*), bovine (*C*), and porcine (*D*) thyroid gland

The inset to *D* illustrates the subtracheal connection in transverse section
in the pig.

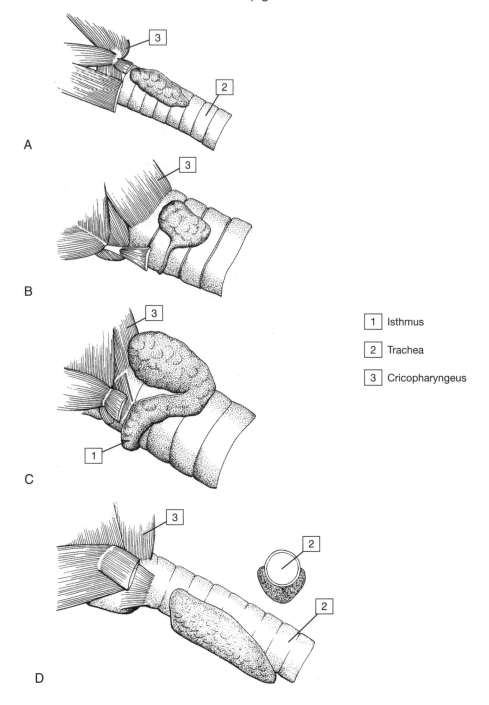

A

B

C

D

1	Isthmus
2	Trachea
3	Cricopharyngeus

THE THORAX

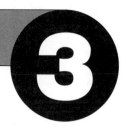

3

Figure 3-1 Schema of canine circulation

Vessels carrying oxygenated blood are shown in white, those carrying deoxygenated blood in black.

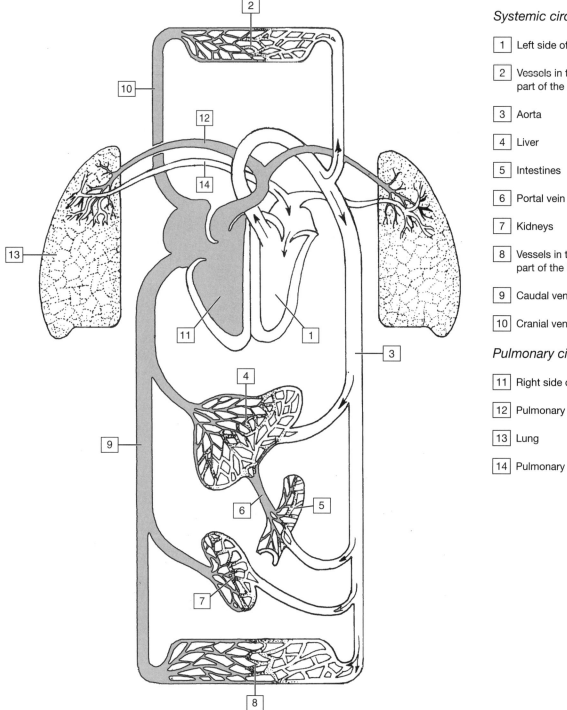

Systemic circulation:

1 Left side of the heart

2 Vessels in the cranial part of the body

3 Aorta

4 Liver

5 Intestines

6 Portal vein

7 Kidneys

8 Vessels in the caudal part of the body

9 Caudal vena cava

10 Cranial vena cava

Pulmonary circulation:

11 Right side of the heart

12 Pulmonary artery

13 Lung

14 Pulmonary vein

Figure 3-2 Canine trunk muscles, deeper layers

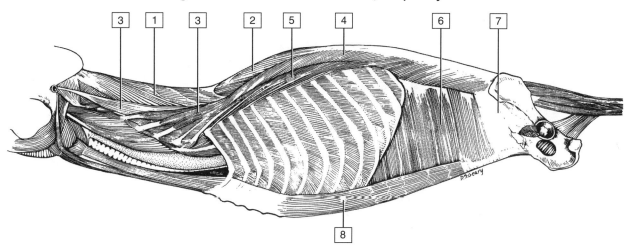

1	Semispinalis capitis	5	Iliocostalis
2	Spinalis et semispinalis	6	Transversus abdominis
3	Longissimus capitis and cervicis	7	Transverse fascia
4	Longissimus thoracis	8	Rectus abdominis

Figure 3-3   Canine trunk muscles, deepest layers

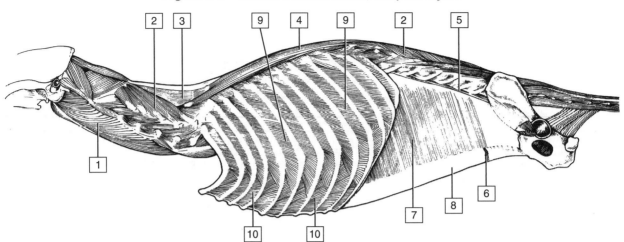

1 Longus capitis	6 Rectus abdominis
2 Multifidus	7 Transversus abdominis
3 Spinalis cervicis	8 Aponeurosis of transversus abdominis
4 Spinalis et semispinalis	9 External intercostal muscles
5 Quadratus lumborum	10 Internal intercostal muscles

Saunders Veterinary Anatomy Coloring Book

Figure 3-4   Muscular suspension of the canine thorax between the forelimbs

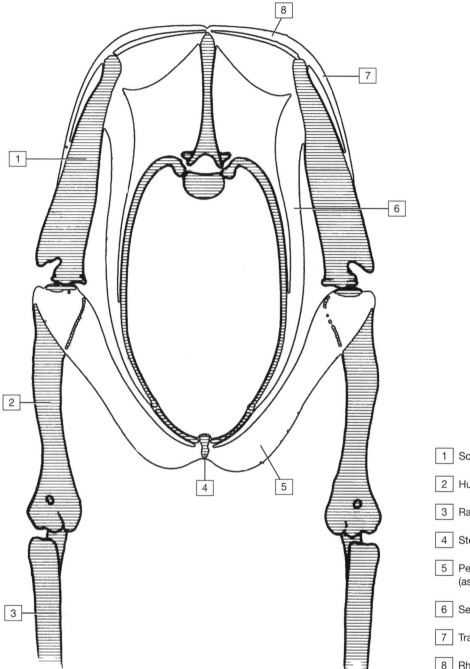

1	Scapula
2	Humerus
3	Radius and ulna
4	Sternum
5	Pectoralis profundus (ascendens)
6	Serratus ventralis
7	Trapezius
8	Rhomboideus

Figure 3-5   The distribution of the canine pleura and pericardium

The heavy lines indicate the pleura.

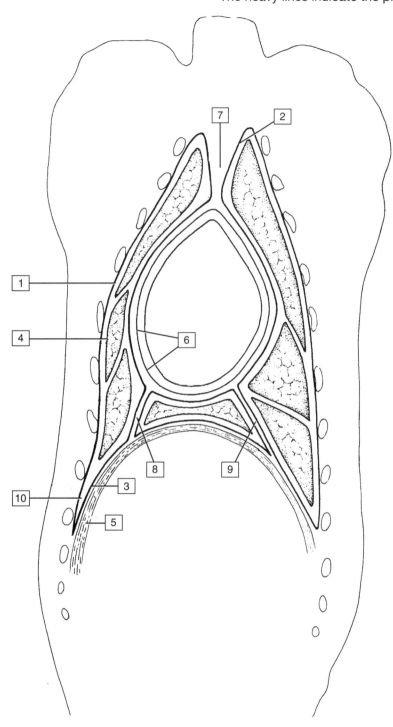

1	Costal pleura
2	Mediastinal pleura
3	Diaphragmatic pleura
4	Visceral pleura
5	Diaphragm
6	Parietal pericardium; its outer fibrous layer tightly adheres to its inner serous layer
7	Cranial mediastinum
8	Caudal mediastinum
8′	Cupula pleurae
9	Plica venae cavae
10	Costodiaphragmatic recess

Figure 3-6 Section of the canine heart exposing the four chambers

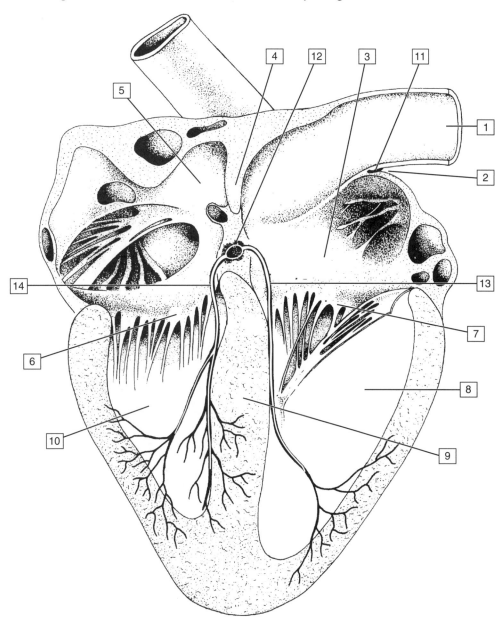

1	Cranial vena cava	8	Right ventricle
2	Terminal sulcus	9	Interventricular septum
3	Right atrium	10	Left ventricle
4	Interatrial septum	11	Sinoatrial node
5	Left atrium	12	Atrioventricular node
6	Left atrioventricular valve	13	Right and left limbs of atrioventricular bundle
7	Right atrioventricular valve	14	Right and left limbs of atrioventricular bundle

Figure 3-7   Canine pericardium

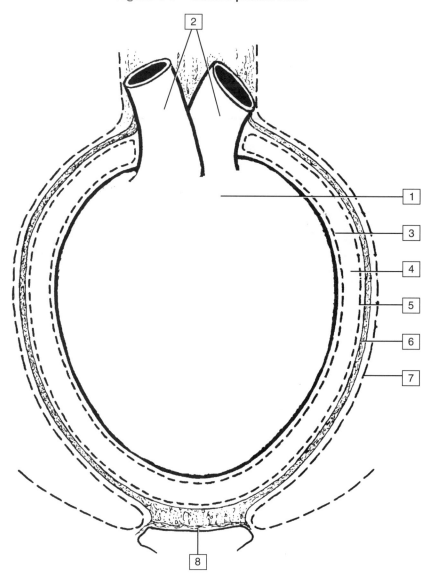

1 Heart	5 Parietal pericardium
2 Great vessels	6 Connective tissue layer of the parietal pericardium
3 Visceral pericardium (epicardium)	7 Mediastinal pleura
4 Pericardial cavity (exaggerated in size)	8 Sternopericardial ligament

Figure 3-8   Canine cardiac nerves and related ganglia, left lateral view

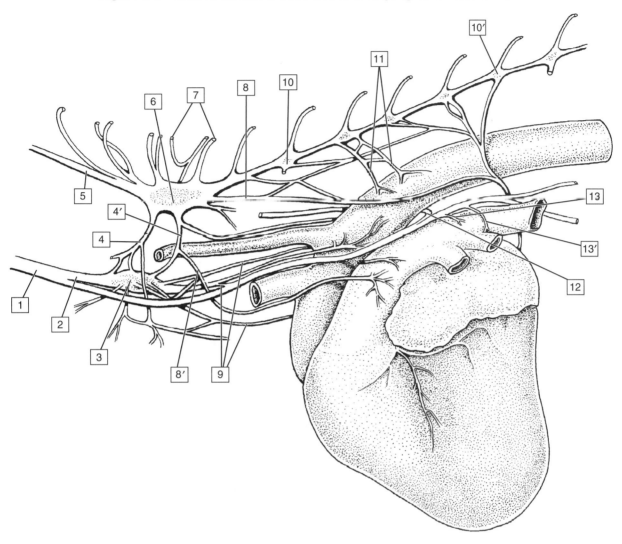

1	Vagosympathetic trunk	8'	Caudodorsal and caudoventral cervicothoracic cardiac n.
2	Sympathetic trunk	9	Vertebral cardiac n.
3	Middle cervical ganglion	10	Third and seventh thoracic ganglia
4	Cranial and caudal limbs of ansa subclavia	10'	Third and seventh thoracic ganglia
4'	Cranial and caudal limbs of ansa subclavia	11	Thoracic cardiac n.
5	Vertebral n.	12	Left recurrent laryngeal n.
6	Cervicothoracic ganglion	13	Cranial and caudal vagal cardiac n.
7	Communicating branches	13'	Cranial and caudal vagal cardiac n.
8	Caudodorsal and caudoventral cervicothoracic cardiac n.		

Figure 3-9 The components of the canine arterial wall

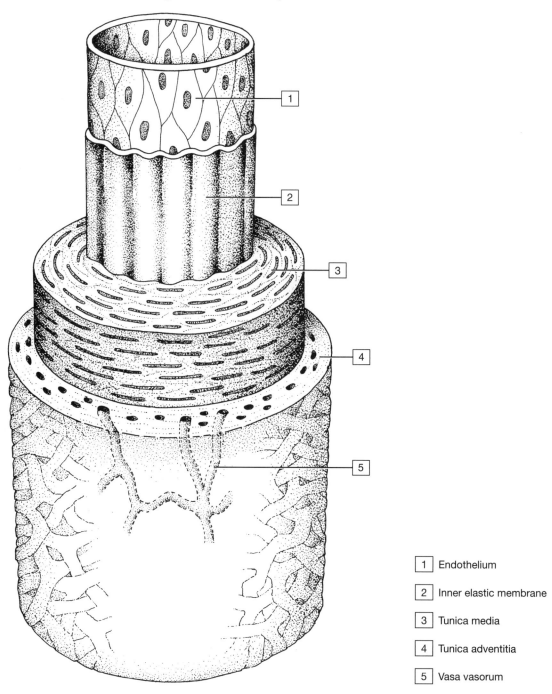

1 Endothelium

2 Inner elastic membrane

3 Tunica media

4 Tunica adventitia

5 Vasa vasorum

Figure 3-10   Branching of the canine aortic arch

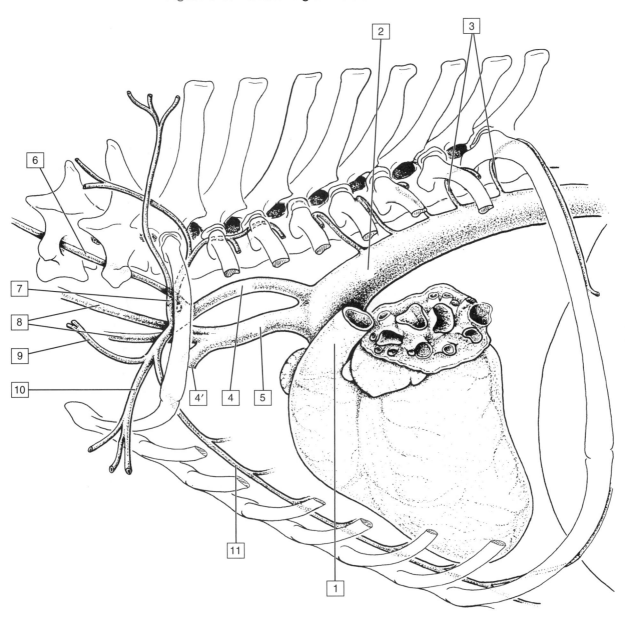

1 Pulmonary trunk	6 Vertebral a.
2 Aorta	7 Costocervical trunk
3 Intercostal aa.	8 Left and right common carotid aa.
4 Left subclavian a.	9 Superficial cervical a.
4' Right subclavian a.	10 Axillary a.
5 Brachiocephalic trunk	11 Internal thoracic a.

Figure 3-11   Diagrams of the canine fetal (*A*) and postnatal
(*B*) circulatory systems

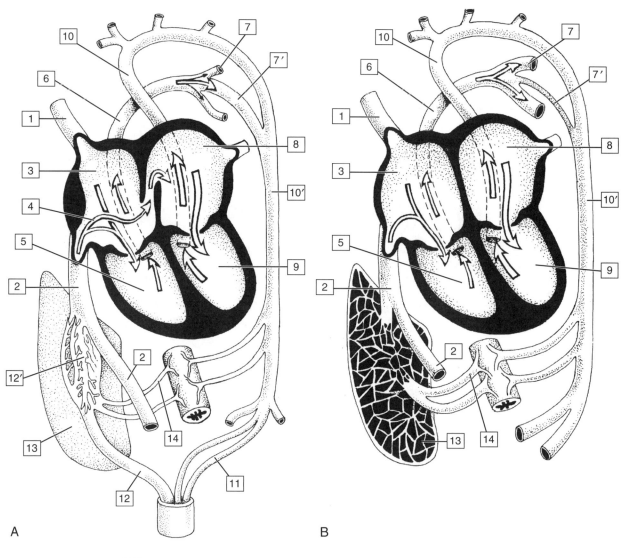

A

B

1 Cranial vena cava	9 Left ventricle
2 Caudal vena cava	10 Aortic arch
3 Right atrium	10′ Descending aorta
4 Arrow entering oval foramen	11 Umbilical artery
5 Right ventricle	12 Umbilical vein
6 Pulmonary trunk	12′ Ductus venosus
7 Pulmonary artery	13 Liver
7′ Ductus arteriosus (in *B*, vestige)	14 Portal vein
8 Left atrium	

Figure 3-12   Lymph drainage of the canine lumbosacral area, ventral view

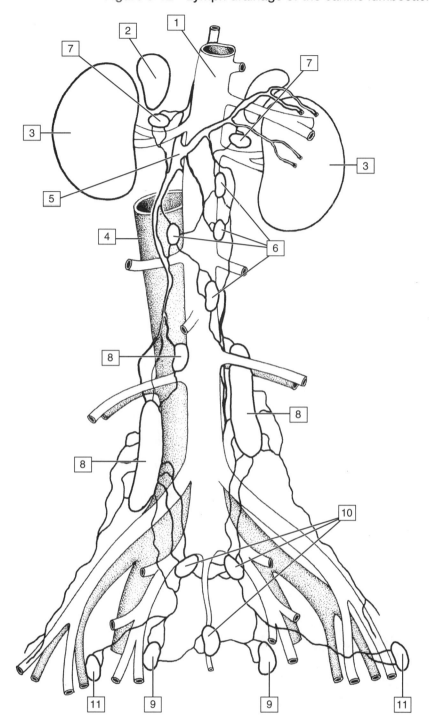

1	Aorta
2	Adrenals
3	Kidneys
4	Caudal vena cava
5	Cisterna chyli
6	Lumbar aortic nodes
7	Renal nodes
8	Medial iliac nodes
9	Hypogastric nodes
10	Sacral nodes
11	Deep inguinal (iliofemoral) nodes

Figure 3-13   The vessels on the floor of the canine thorax

The transversus thoracis has been removed on the right.

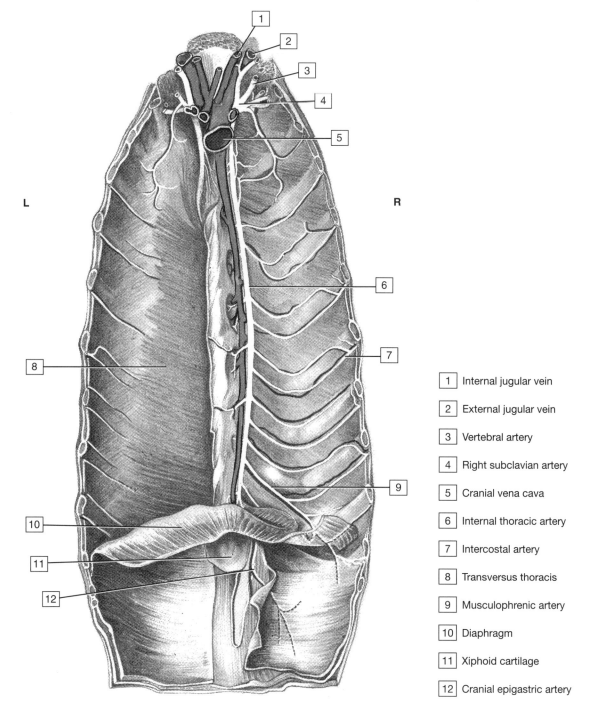

1	Internal jugular vein
2	External jugular vein
3	Vertebral artery
4	Right subclavian artery
5	Cranial vena cava
6	Internal thoracic artery
7	Intercostal artery
8	Transversus thoracis
9	Musculophrenic artery
10	Diaphragm
11	Xiphoid cartilage
12	Cranial epigastric artery

L

R

Saunders Veterinary Anatomy Coloring Book
Copyright © 2011 by Saunders, an imprint of Elsevier Inc.

Figure 3-14   Muscles of the canine neck and thorax, lateral view

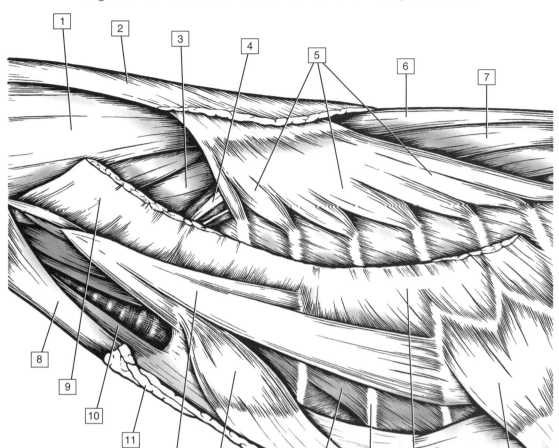

1	Splenius	8	Sternocephalicus	15	External intercostal muscle III
2	Rhomboideus	9	Serratus ventralis (cervicis)	16	4th rib
3	Longissimus cervicis	10	Sternothyroideus	17	Serratus ventralis (thoracis)
4	Longissimus thoracis	11	Superficial pectoral	18	Rectus abdominis
5	Serratus dorsalis cranialis	12	Scalenus	19	External abdominal oblique
6	Spinalis and semispinalis thoracis	13	Rectus thoracis		
7	Longissimus thoracis	14	Deep pectoral		

Figure 3-15   Left and right surface projections of the feline heart and lung

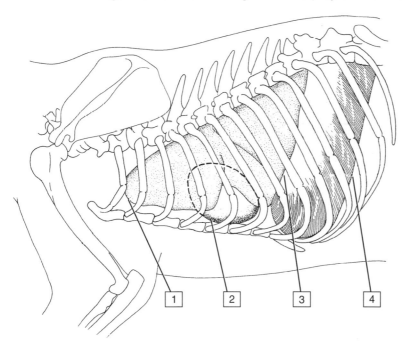

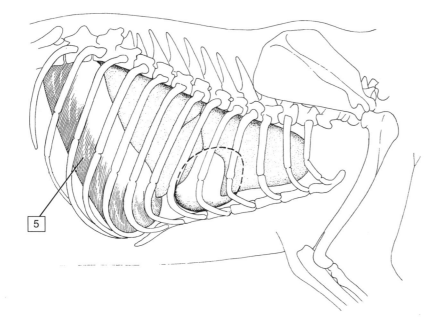

1	Apex of left lung
2	Heart
3	Basal border of lung
4	Line of pleural reflection
5	Diaphragm

Figure 3-16   Projections of the equine heart and lung on the left and
right thoracic walls

The heavy line indicates the caudal border of the triceps.

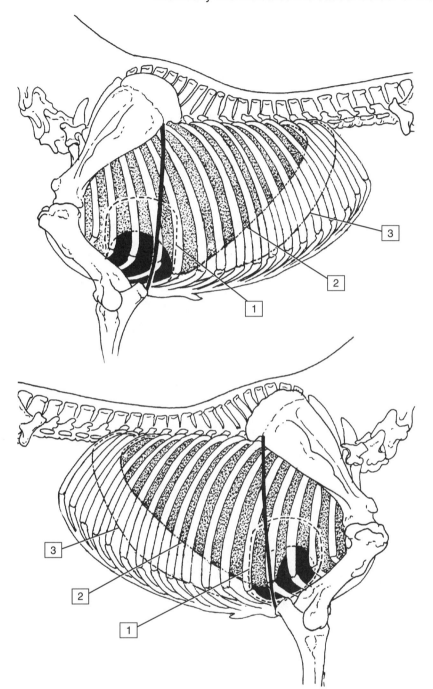

1	Outline of heart
2	Basal border of lung
3	Line of pleural reflection

Figure 3-17   Left lateral view of the bovine thoracic cavity

The left lung and part of the mediastinal pleura have been removed.

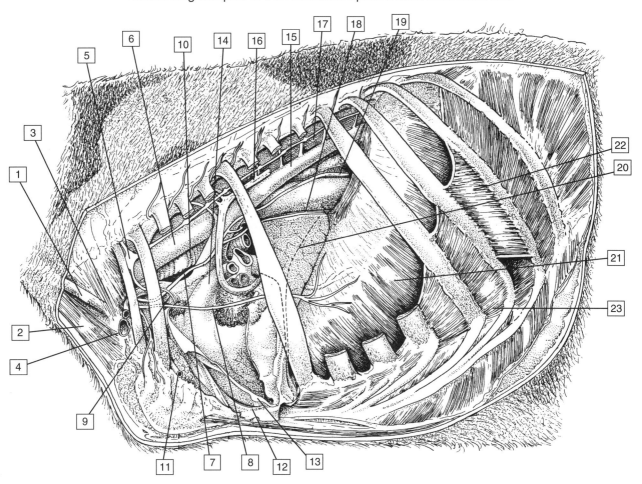

1	External jugular vein	9	One of the cardiac nerves	17	Greater splanchnic nerve
2	Sternocephalicus	10	Trachea	18	Ventral vagal trunk
3	Axillary artery	11	Internal thoracic artery	19	Dorsal vagal trunk
4	Axillary vein	12	Mediastinal pleura	20	Cranial extent of diaphragm
5	Cervicothoracic ganglion	13	Pericardium, reflected	21	Diaphragm
6	Esophagus	14	Pulmonary trunk	22	Internal intercostal muscle
7	Vagus	15	Aorta	23	External intercostal muscle
8	Phrenic nerve	16	Left azygous vein		

Figure 3-18   Lobation and bronchial tree of the bovine lungs,
schematic dorsal view

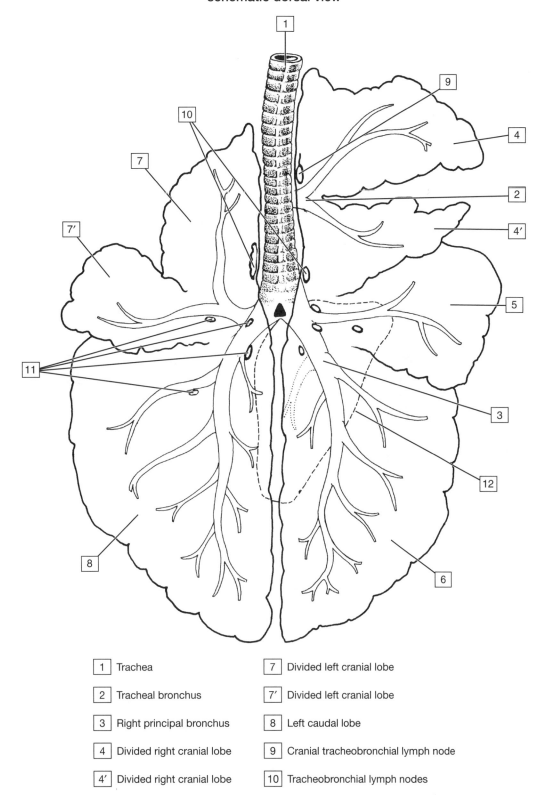

1	Trachea	7	Divided left cranial lobe
2	Tracheal bronchus	7'	Divided left cranial lobe
3	Right principal bronchus	8	Left caudal lobe
4	Divided right cranial lobe	9	Cranial tracheobronchial lymph node
4'	Divided right cranial lobe	10	Tracheobronchial lymph nodes
5	Middle lobe	11	Pulmonary lymph nodes
6	Right caudal lobe	12	Outline of accessory lobe of right lung

Figure 3-19   Porcine embryo after fusion of the endocardial tube

A, Ventral view of the cranial part of a 15-day-old pig embryo after fusion of the endocardial tube. *B,* Transverse section of a seven- to eight-somite embryo taken at the level of 5.

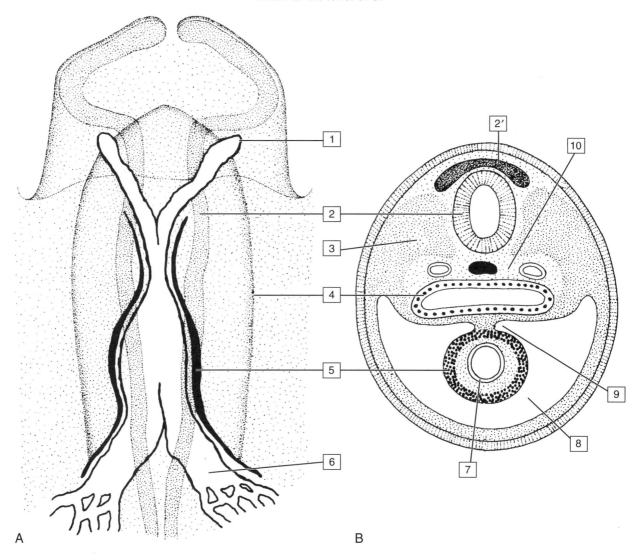

A

B

1	First aortic arch		6	Vitelline vein
2	Neural tube		7	Endocardial tube
2'	Neural crest		8	Pericardial cavity
3	Somite		9	Dorsal mesocardium
4	Foregut		10	Notochord and dorsal aortae
5	Epimyocardial wall of the fused endocardial tubes			

Figure 3-20   Porcine heart in situ

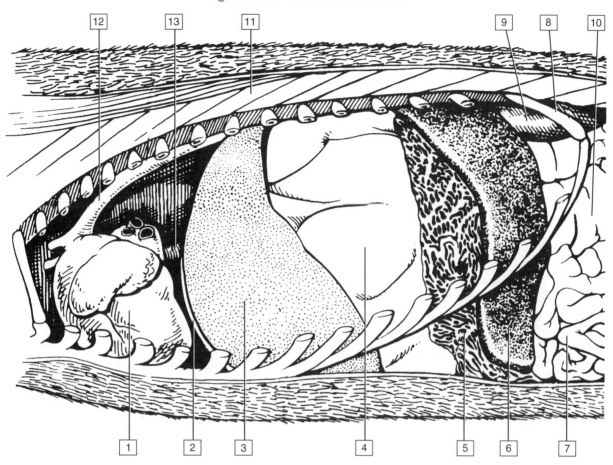

1 Heart	8 Last rib
2 Diaphragm	9 Left kidney
3 Left lobe of liver	10 Ascending colon
4 Stomach, greatly dilated	11 Back muscles
5 Greater omentum, gastrosplenic ligament	12 Aorta
6 Spleen	13 Caudal vena cava
7 Jejunum	

Figure 3-21   Porcine lymph centers of the thorax, left lateral view

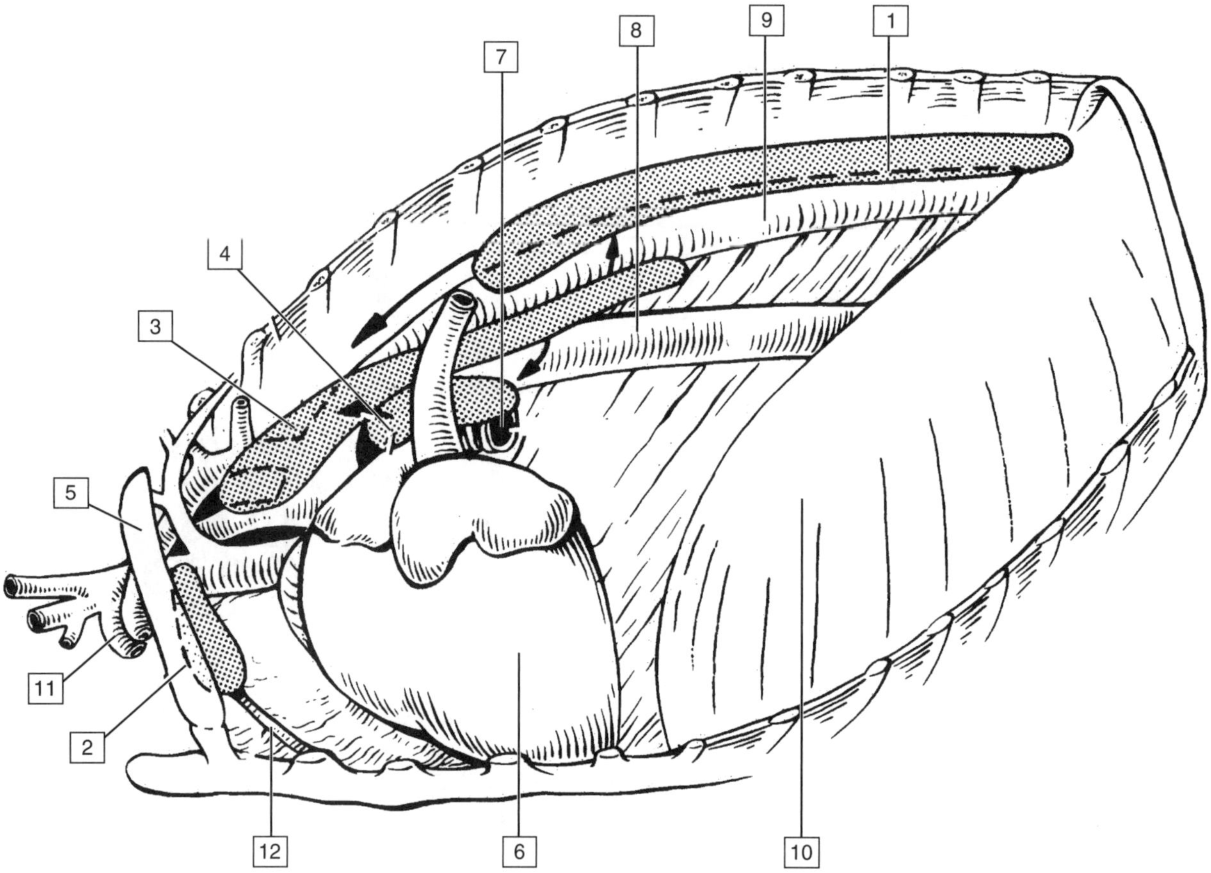

1	Dorsal thoracic lymph center	8	Esophagus
2	Ventral thoracic lymph center	9	Aorta
3	Mediastinal lymph center	10	Diaphragm
4	Tracheobronchial lymph center	11	Axillary vein and artery
5	First rib	12	Internal thoracic artery
6	Heart		
7	Left bronchus		

Figure 3-22   Avian flight muscles, dissected and shown in ventral view

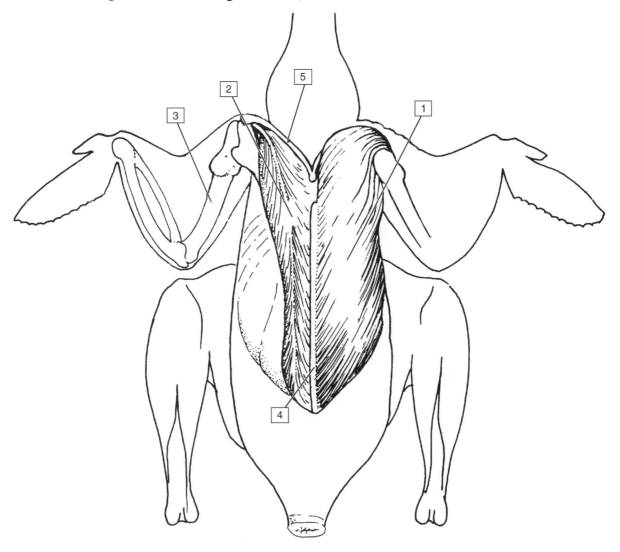

1	Pectoralis
2	Supracoracoideus
3	Humerus
4	Sternum
5	Clavicle

Figure 3-23   Right avian lung (medioventral view) and related air sacs

The intrapulmonic structures have been simplified.

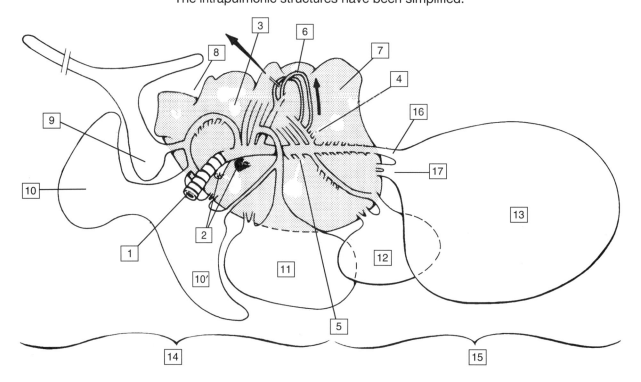

1 Primary bronchus	10 Extra- and intrathoracic parts of clavicular air sac
2 Pulmonary vessels at hilus	10′ Extra- and intrathoracic parts of clavicular air sac
3 Medioventral bronchi	11 Cranial thoracic air sac
4 Mediodorsal bronchi	12 Caudal thoracic air sac
5 Lateroventral bronchi	13 Abdominal air sac
6 Loops of parabronchi	14 Cranial air sacs, functionally related to paleopulmonic parabronchi
7 Lung	15 Caudal air sacs, functionally related to neopulmonic parabronchi
8 Indentations caused by ribs	16 Direct (saccobronchial) connection
9 Cervical air sac	17 Indirect (recurrent bronchial) connection of air sac to lung

Saunders Veterinary Anatomy Coloring Book
Copyright © 2011 by Saunders, an imprint of Elsevier Inc.

Figure 3-24   Ventral view of the avian kidneys, and vessels and nerves in their vicinity

The right kidney shows the branches of the ureter; the left, the renal vessels.
Cranial (*A*), middle (*B*), and caudal (*C*) divisions of kidney.

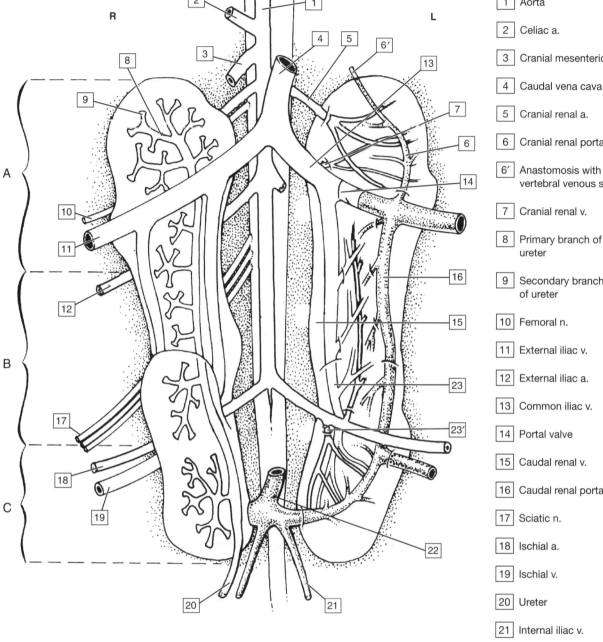

1	Aorta
2	Celiac a.
3	Cranial mesenteric a.
4	Caudal vena cava
5	Cranial renal a.
6	Cranial renal portal v.
6'	Anastomosis with vertebral venous sinus
7	Cranial renal v.
8	Primary branch of ureter
9	Secondary branch of ureter
10	Femoral n.
11	External iliac v.
12	External iliac a.
13	Common iliac v.
14	Portal valve
15	Caudal renal v.
16	Caudal renal portal v.
17	Sciatic n.
18	Ischial a.
19	Ischial v.
20	Ureter
21	Internal iliac v.
22	Caudal mesenteric v.
23	Middle renal a.
23'	Caudal renal a.

THE ABDOMEN

Figure 4-1 Rectus sheath of the canine in transverse sections

A, Cranial and *B,* caudal to the umbilicus and near the pubis, *C.*

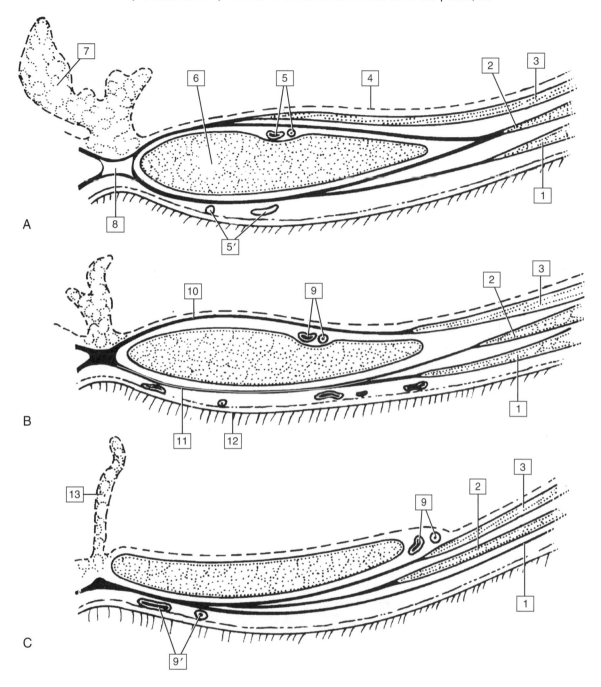

1 External abdominal oblique	**5'** Cranial superficial epigastric vessels	**9'** Caudal superficial epigastric vessels
2 Internal abdominal oblique	**6** Rectus abdominis	**10** Internal lamina of rectus sheath
3 Transversus abdominis	**7** Fat-filled falciform ligament	**11** External lamina of rectus sheath
4 Peritoneum	**8** Linea alba	**12** Skin
5 Cranial epigastric vessels	**9** Caudal epigastric vessels	**13** Median ligament of the bladder

Figure 4-2   Canine inguinal canal and pelvic diaphragm, left lateral view

The external abdominal oblique muscle has been removed.

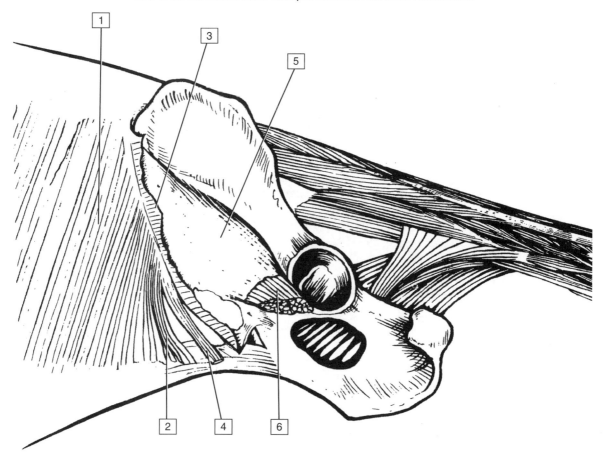

1	Internal abdominal oblique
2	Free caudal edge of internal oblique, forming border of deep inguinal ring
3	Stump of external oblique aponeurosis reflected caudally
4	Cremaster derived from internal oblique
5	Iliac fascia covering iliopsoas
6	Iliopsoas

Figure 4-3   Schematic transverse section through the canine abdomen

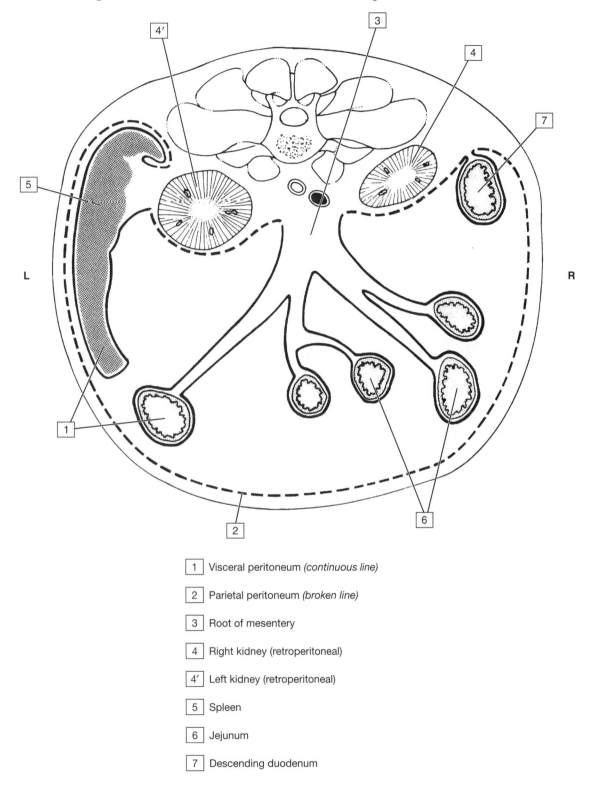

1	Visceral peritoneum *(continuous line)*
2	Parietal peritoneum *(broken line)*
3	Root of mesentery
4	Right kidney (retroperitoneal)
4'	Left kidney (retroperitoneal)
5	Spleen
6	Jejunum
7	Descending duodenum

Figure 4-4   Paramedian section of the canine abdominal cavity to show the disposition of the peritoneum

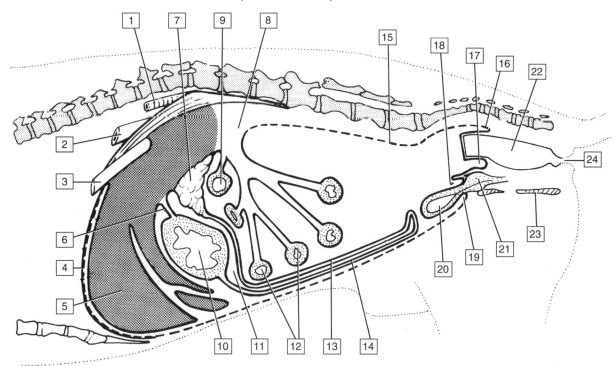

1	Aorta	13	Deep wall of greater omentum
2	Esophagus	14	Superficial wall of greater omentum
3	Caudal vena cava	15	Parietal peritoneum
4	Diaphragm	16	Pararectal fossa
5	Liver	17	Rectogenital pouch
6	Lesser omentum	18	Vesicogenital pouch
7	Pancreas	19	Pubovesical pouch
8	Root of mesentery	20	Bladder
9	Transverse colon	21	Prostate
10	Stomach	22	Rectum
11	Omental bursa	23	Ischium
12	Small intestine	24	Anus

Saunders Veterinary Anatomy Coloring Book
Copyright © 2011 by Saunders, an imprint of Elsevier Inc.

Figure 4-5   Distribution of the canine celiac artery, ventral view

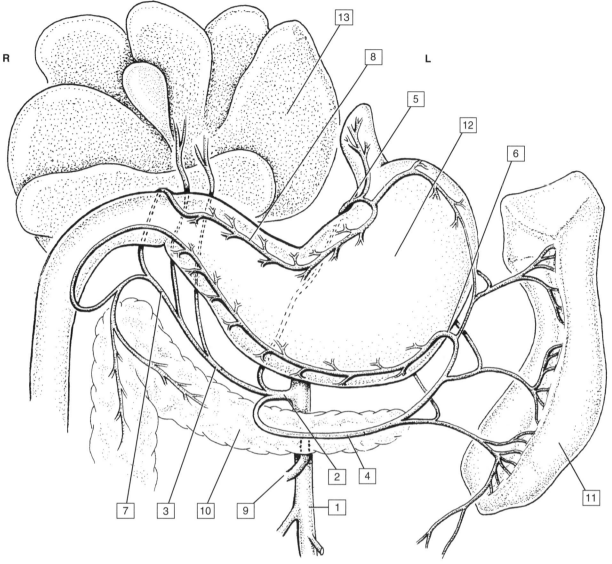

1 Aorta	8 Right gastric artery
2 Celiac artery	9 Cranial mesenteric artery
3 Hepatic artery	10 Pancreas
4 Splenic artery	11 Spleen
5 Left gastric artery	12 Stomach
6 Left gastroepiploic artery	13 Liver
7 Gastroduodenal artery	

Figure 4-6   Canine abdominal organs after removal of the greater omentum,
ventral view

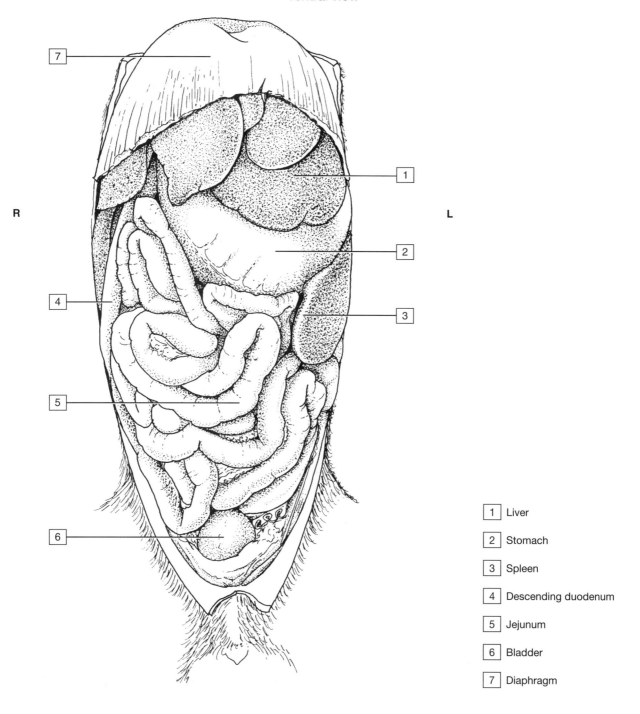

1	Liver
2	Stomach
3	Spleen
4	Descending duodenum
5	Jejunum
6	Bladder
7	Diaphragm

Figure 4-7   Muscles of the canine perineal region

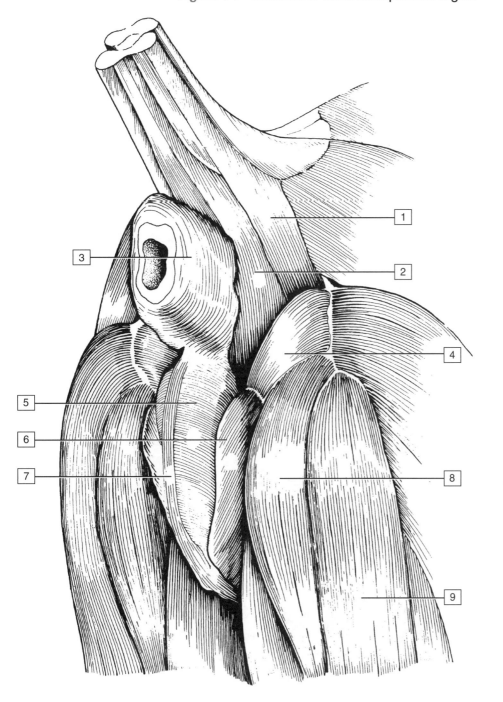

1   Coccygeus

2   Levator ani

3   External anal sphincter

4   Internal obturator

5   Bulbospongiosus

6   Ischiocavernosus

7   Retractor penis

8   Semimembranosus

9   Semitendinosus

Figure 4-8   Distribution of the canine cranial and caudal mesenteric arteries
to the intestines, dorsal view

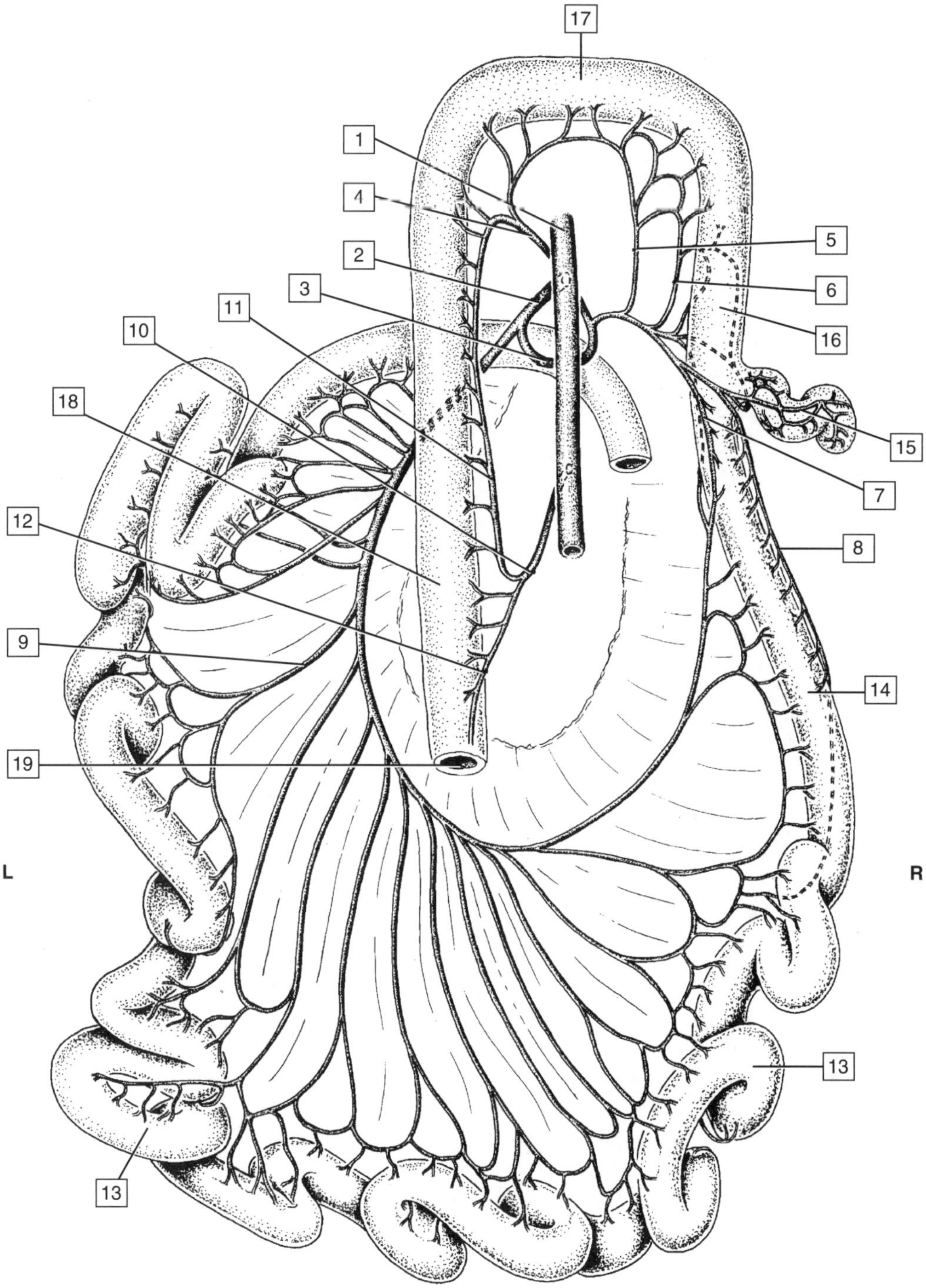

1	Aorta	6	Colic branch of ileocolic artery	11	Left colic artery	16	Ascending colon
2	Cranial mesenteric artery	7	Mesenteric ileal branch	12	Cranial rectal artery	17	Transverse colon
3	Ileocolic artery	8	Antimesenteric ileal branch	13	Jejunum	18	Descending colon
4	Middle colic artery	9	Jejunal arteries	14	Ileum	19	Rectum
5	Right colic artery	10	Caudal mesenteric artery	15	Cecum		

Figure 4-9   Semischematic dorsal view of the formation of the canine portal vein

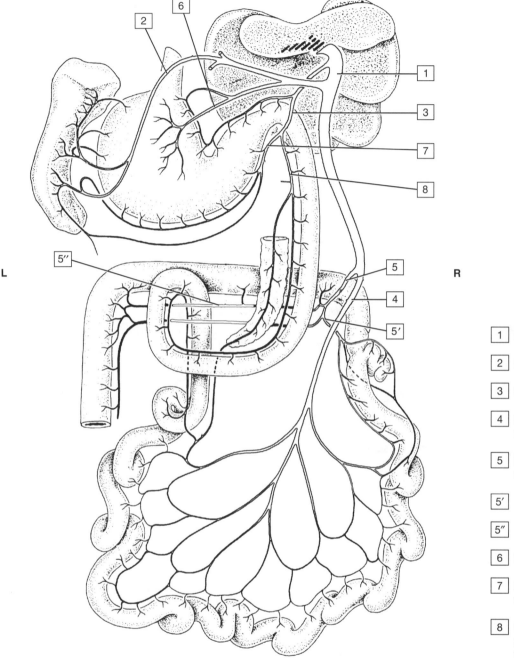

L

R

1 Portal vein

2 Splenic vein

3 Gastroduodenal vein

4 Cranial mesenteric vein

5 Caudal mesenteric vein

5′ Ileocolic vein

5″ Middle colic vein

6 Left gastric vein

7 Right gastroepiploic vein

8 Cranial pancreaticoduodenal vein

Figure 4-10   Visceral surface of the canine liver

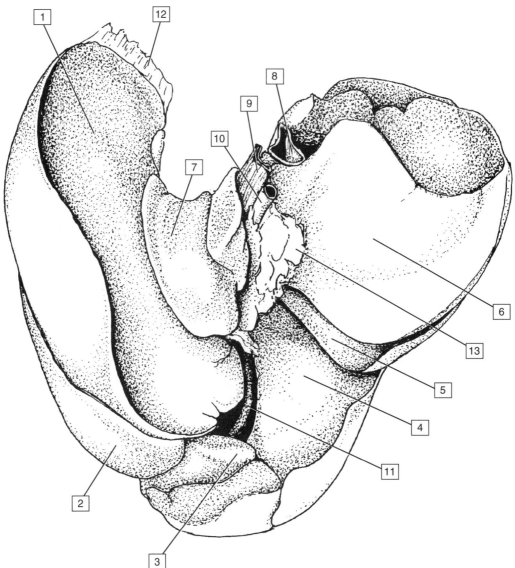

1	Left lateral lobe	8	Caudal vena cava
2	Left medial lobe	9	Portal vein
3	Quadrate lobe	10	Hepatic artery
4	Right medial lobe	11	Gallbladder
5	Right lateral lobe	12	Left triangular ligament
6	Caudate process (of caudate lobe)	13	Lesser omentum
7	Papillary process (of caudate lobe)		

Figure 4-11   Development of the canine liver

A, Early development: a cranial branch of the endodermal diverticulum invades the septum transversum; a caudal branch forms the gallbladder and cystic duct. *B,* A later stage, in which the developing liver expands caudally into the abdominal cavity.

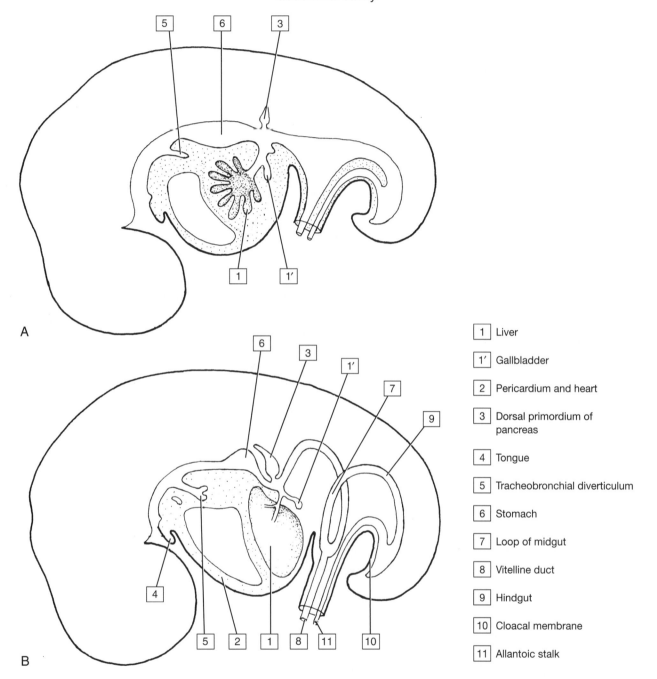

1 | Liver
1' | Gallbladder
2 | Pericardium and heart
3 | Dorsal primordium of pancreas
4 | Tongue
5 | Tracheobronchial diverticulum
6 | Stomach
7 | Loop of midgut
8 | Vitelline duct
9 | Hindgut
10 | Cloacal membrane
11 | Allantoic stalk

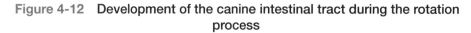

Figure 4-12 Development of the canine intestinal tract during the rotation process

The midgut loop is herniated into the extraembryonic celom.

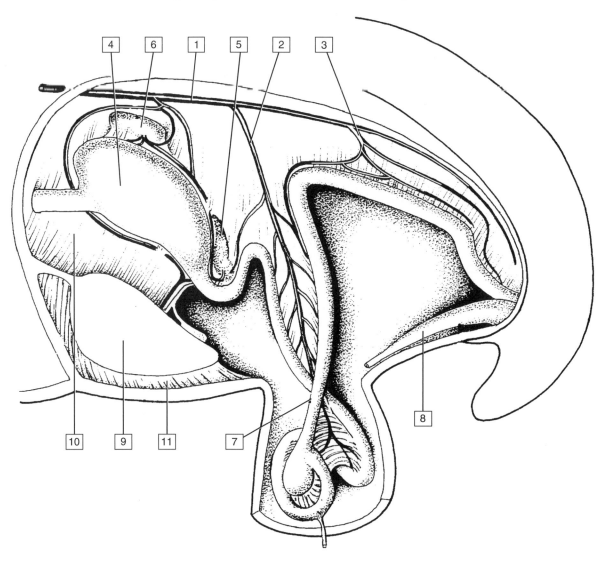

1	Celiac artery	7	Loop of midgut
2	Cranial mesenteric artery	8	Bladder expansion of the urogenital sinus
3	Caudal mesenteric artery	9	Liver
4	Stomach	10	Lesser omentum
5	Pancreas	11	Falciform ligament
6	Spleen		

Figure 4-13 Lymph drainage from the organs in the canine abdominal and pelvic cavities

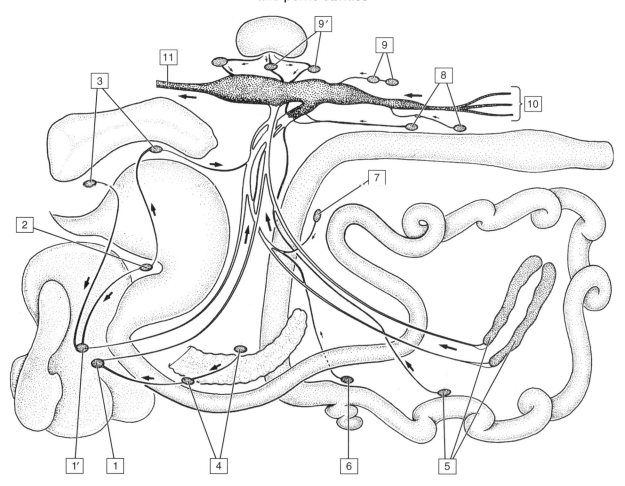

1 Right hepatic node	7 Middle colic node
1' Left hepatic node	8 Caudal mesenteric nodes
2 Gastric node	9 Lumbar aortic nodes
3 Splenic nodes	9' Renal nodes
4 Pancreaticoduodenal nodes	10 Efferents from the iliosacral region
5 Jejunal nodes	11 Continuation of cisterna chyli as thoracic duct
6 Right colic node	

Figure 4-14   Ganglia and plexuses of the canine abdominal cavity, ventral
view

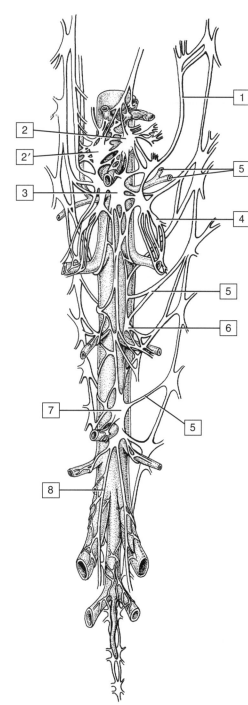

1   Greater splanchnic n.

2   Left celiac ganglion

2' Right celiac ganglion

3   Cranial mesenteric ganglion

4   Renal ganglion

5   Lumbar splanchnic n.

6   Gonadal ganglion

7   Caudal mesenteric ganglion

8   Right hypogastric n.

Figure 4-15   Transverse section of the canine trunk at the level of the 11th thoracic vertebra

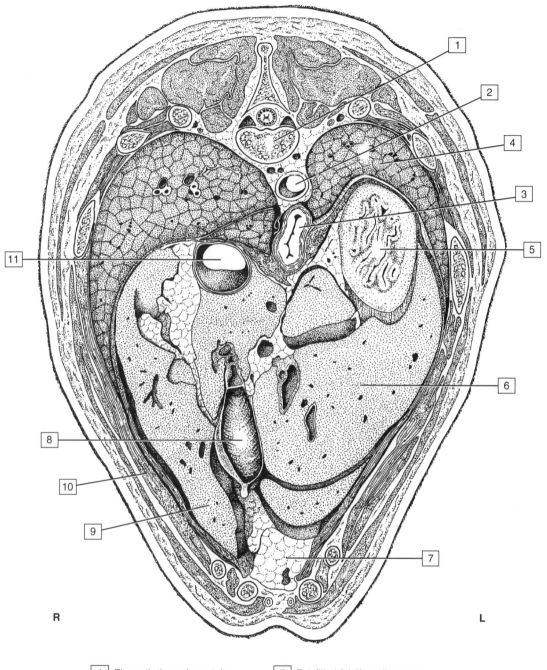

R   L

1	Eleventh thoracic vertebra	7	Fat-filled falciform ligament
2	Aorta	8	Gallbladder
3	Esophagus	9	Right medial lobe of liver
4	Left lung	10	Diaphragm
5	Fundus of stomach	11	Caudal vena cava
6	Left lateral lobe of liver		

Figure 4-16   Transverse section of the canine trunk at the level of the 12th
thoracic vertebra

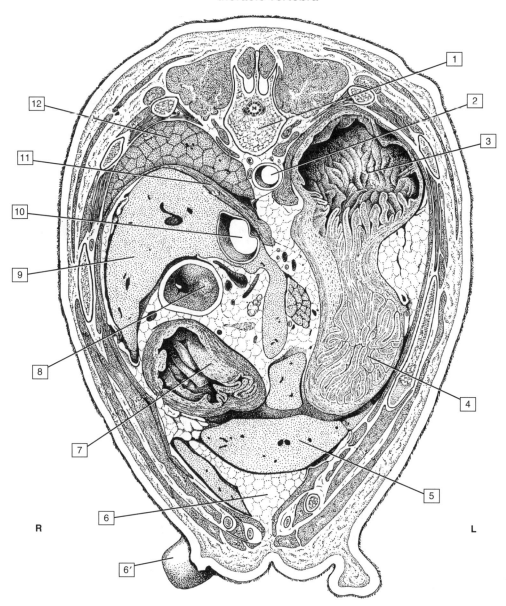

R   L

1	Twelfth thoracic vertebra	6	Fat-filled falciform ligament	10	Caudal vena cava
2	Aorta	6′	Teat	11	Diaphragm
3	Fundus of stomach	7	Pyloric part of stomach	12	Right lung
4	Body of stomach	8	Descending duodenum		
5	Liver	9	Caudate process of liver		

Saunders Veterinary Anatomy Coloring Book

Figure 4-17   Transverse sections of the canine abdomen at the level of the first lumbar vertebra (A) and fourth or fifth lumbar vertebra (B)

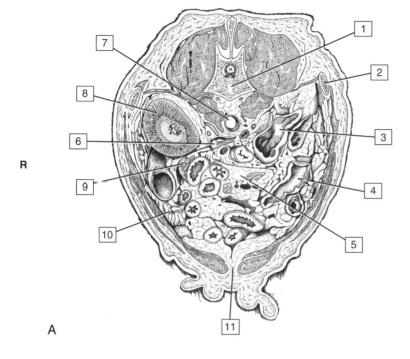

R   L

A

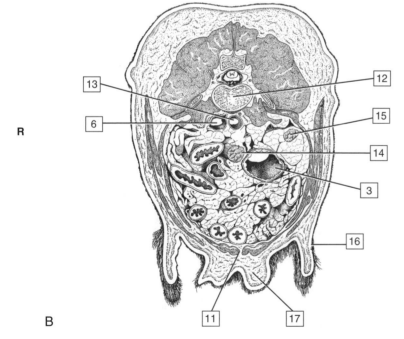

R   L

B

1   First lumbar vertebra

2   Last rib

3   Descending colon

4   Transverse colon

5   Lymph nodes and blood vessels in mesentery; ventral to them is the jejunum

6   Caudal vena cava

7   Aorta, between crura of diaphragm

8   Right kidney

9   Descending duodenum and pancreas

10 Greater omentum

11 Linea alba

12 Lumbar vertebra

13 Aorta

14 Right uterine horn

15 Left uterine horn

16 Flank fold

17 Mammary gland

Figure 4-18   The blood supply of the canine intestinal tract, ventral view

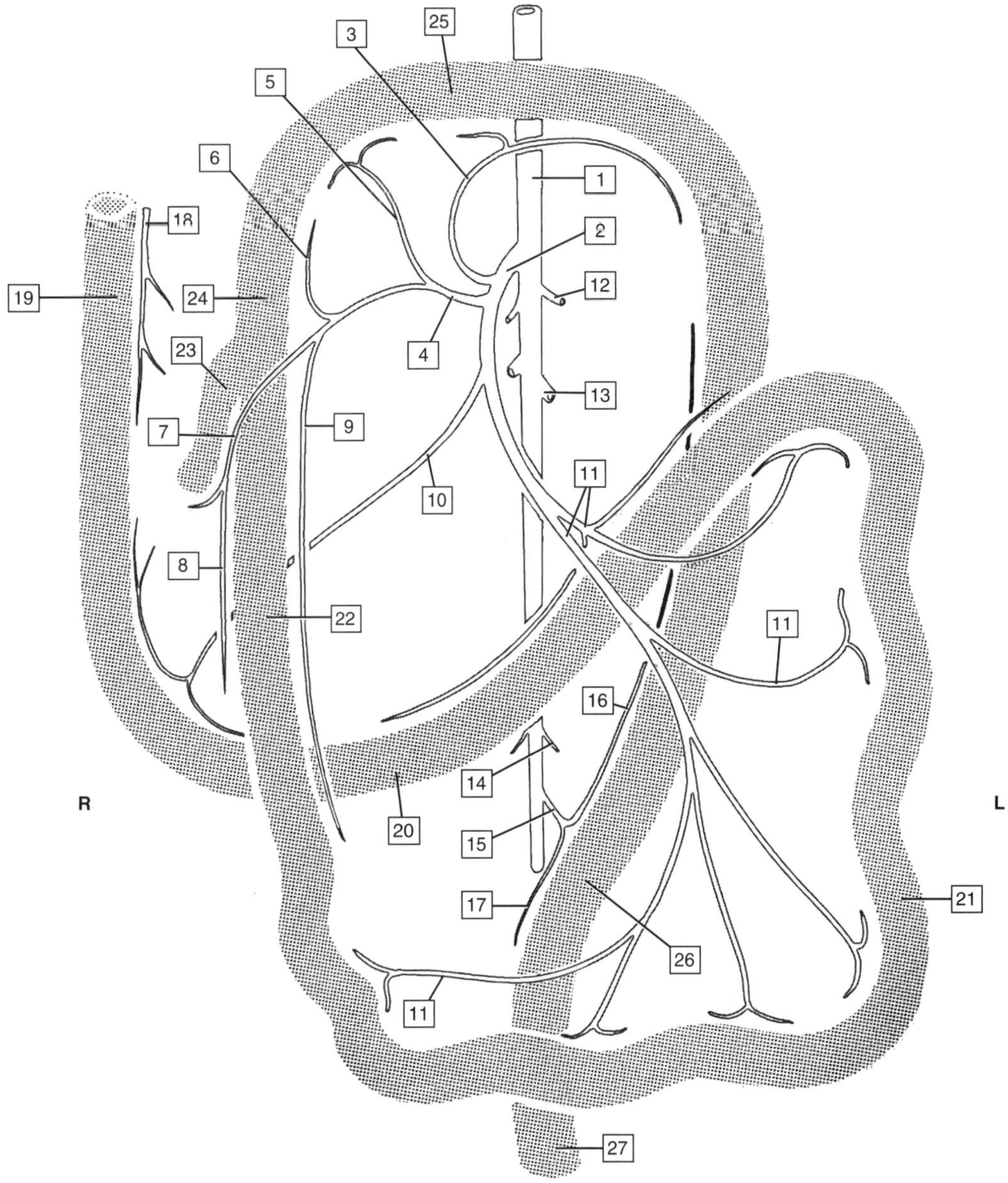

1 Abdominal aorta	8 Antimesenteric ileal branch	13 Renal a.	20 Ascending duodenum
2 Cranial mesenteric a.	9 Mesenteric ileal branch	14 Testicular (ovarian) aa.	21 Jejunum
3 Middle colic a.		15 Caudal mesenteric aa.	22 Ileum
4 Ileocolic a.	10 Caudal pancreaticoduodenal a.	16 Left colic a.	23 Cecum
5 Right colic a.		17 Cranial rectal a.	24 Ascending colon
6 Colic branch of ileocolic a.	11 Jejunal aa.	18 Cranial pancreaticoduodenal a.	25 Transverse colon
7 Cecal a.	12 Phrenicoabdominal aa.	19 Descending duodenum	26 Descending colon
			27 Rectum

Saunders Veterinary Anatomy Coloring Book
Copyright © 2011 by Saunders, an imprint of Elsevier Inc.

Figure 4-19   Canine abdominal muscles and inguinal region of the male,
deep dissection, left side

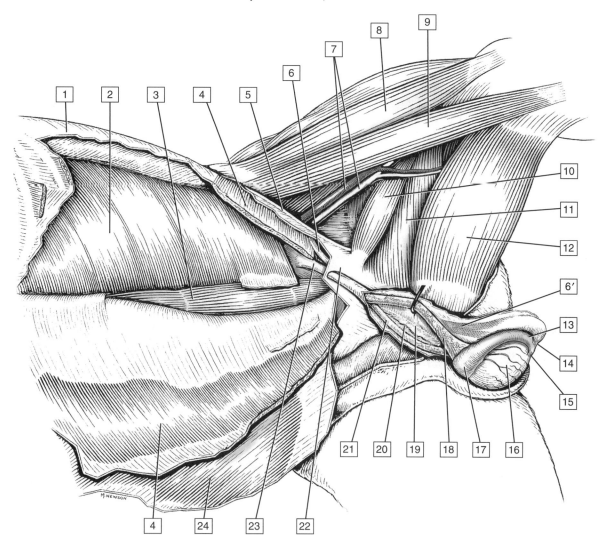

| 1 | Thoracolumbar fascia | 8 | Cranial part of sartorius | 17 | Head of epididymis |

1 Thoracolumbar fascia

2 Transversus abdominis

3 Rectus abdominis

4 Internal abdominal oblique (transected and reflected)

5 Inguinal ligament (caudal border of aponeurosis of external abdominal oblique muscle)

6 Cremaster muscle at its origin

6′ Cremaster muscle on external surface of parietal layer of vaginal tunic

7 Femoral artery and vein

8 Cranial part of sartorius

9 Caudal part of sartorius

10   Pectineus

11 Adductor

12 Gracilis

13 Tail of epididymis

14 Ligament of tail of epididymis

15 Proper ligament of testis

16 Testis in visceral vaginal tunic

17 Head of epididymis

18 Testicular artery and vein in visceral vaginal tunic (mesorchium)

19 Mesorchium

20 Mesoductus deferens

21 Ductus deferens in visceral vaginal tunic

22 Superficial inguinal ring, lateral crus

23 Parietal vaginal tunic in the inguinal canal

24 External abdominal oblique (reflected)

Figure 4-20   Canine peritoneal reflections, sagittal section

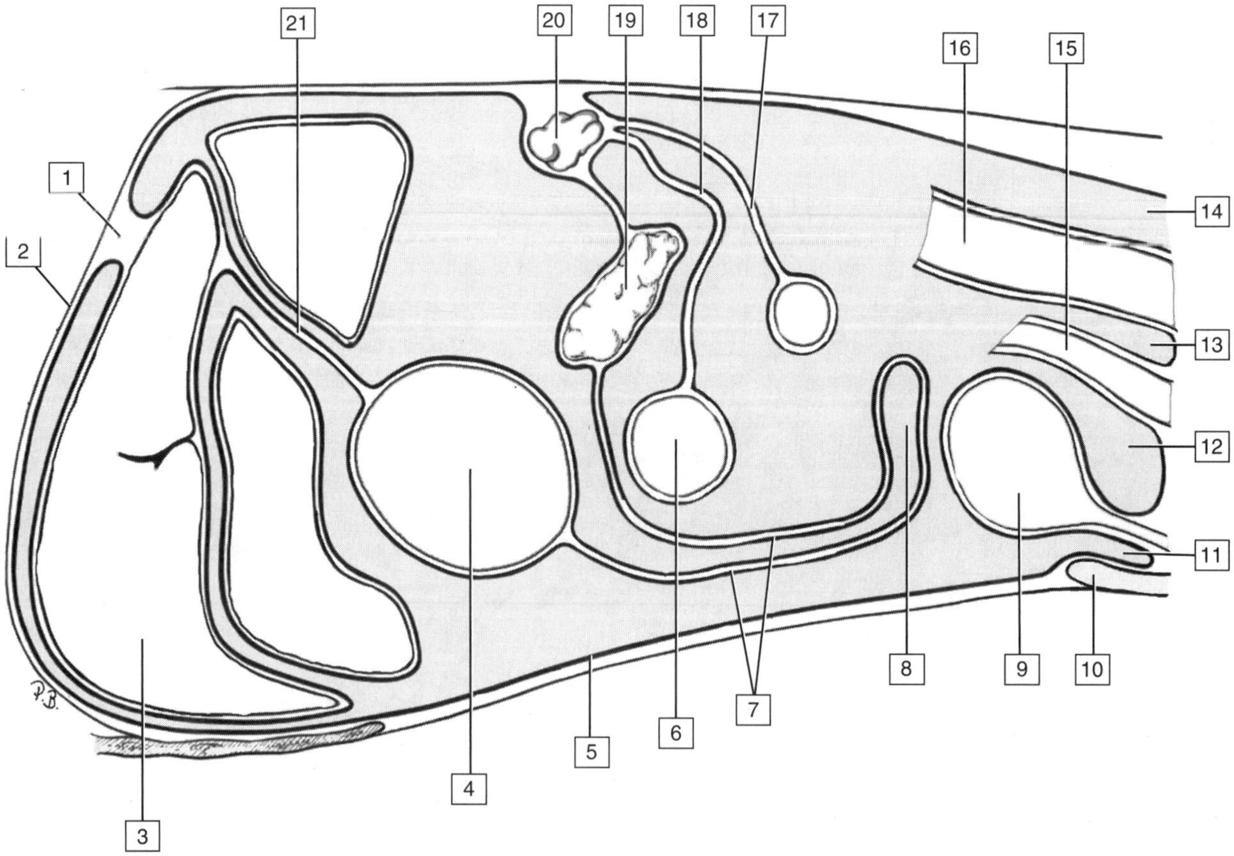

1	Coronary ligament	12	Vesicogenital pouch
2	Diaphragm	13	Rectogenital pouch
3	Liver	14	Pararectal fossa
4	Stomach	15	Uterus
5	Parietal peritoneum	16	Descending colon
6	Transverse colon	17	Mesentery
7	Greater omentum, deep and superficial leaves	18	Transverse mesocolon
8	Omental bursa	19	Left lobe, pancreas
9	Bladder	20	Lymph nodes
10	Symphysis	21	Lesser omentum
11	Pubovesical pouch		

Figure 4-21   Canine liver, visceral aspect

Dog in dorsal recumbency, caudal to cranial view

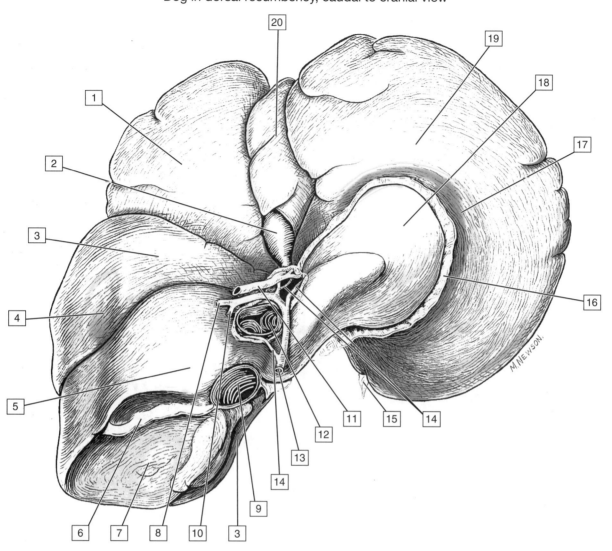

1	Right medial lobe	11	Bile duct
2	Gall bladder	12	Portal vein
3	Right lateral lobe	13	Hepatic artery
4	Duodenal impression	14	Hepatic branch
5	Caudate process of caudate lobe	15	Left triangular ligament
6	Hepatorenal ligament	16	Lesser omentum
7	Renal fossa	17	Gastric impression
8	Gastroduodenal artery	18	Papillary process of caudate lobe
9	Right lateral lobe	19	Left lateral lobe
10	Right gastric artery	20	Caudate lobe

Figure 4-22   Canine branches of celiac and cranial mesenteric arteries with principal anastomoses

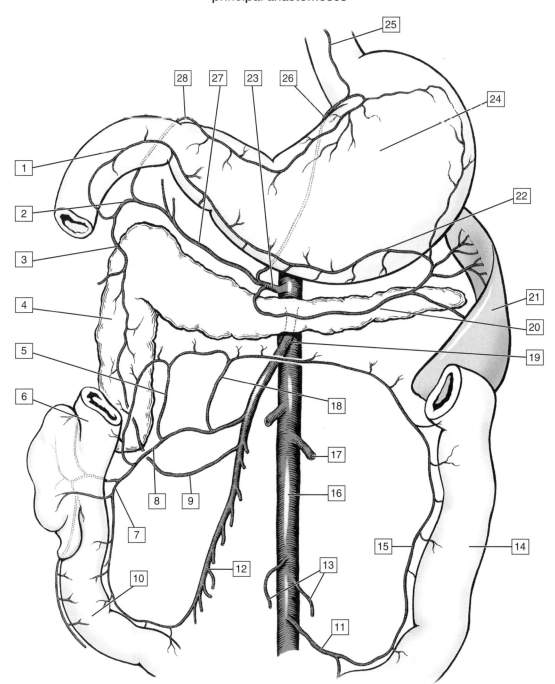

1 Right gastroepiploic	7 Cecal	13 Testicular arteries (ovarian)	18 Middle colic	24 Stomach
2 Gastroduodenal	8 Illiocolic	14 Descending colon	19 Cranial mesenteric	25 Esophageal
3 Cranial pancreaticoduodenal	9 Caudal pancreaticoduodenal	15 Left colic	20 Splenic	26 Left gastric
4 Pancreas	10 Ileum	16 Aorta	21 Spleen	27 Hepatic
5 Right colic	11 Caudal mesenteric	17 Left renal	22 Left gastroepiploic	28 Right gastric
6 Ascending colon	12 Jejunal arteries		23 Celiac	

Figure 4-23   The attachment of the equine abdominal muscles on the pelvis
and the prepubic tendon

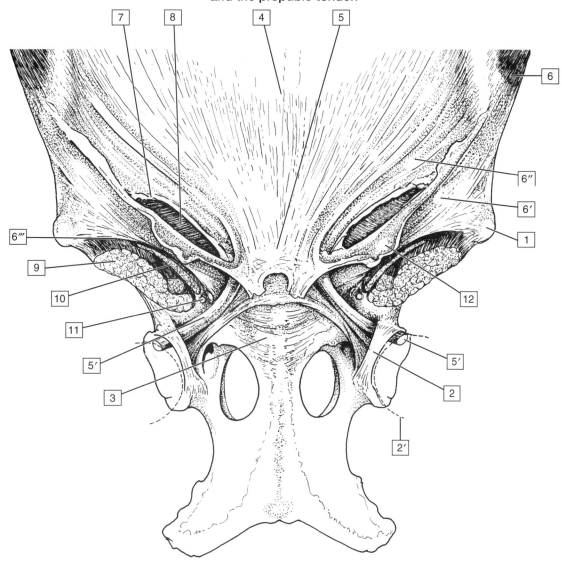

1	Coxal tuber	6″	Abdominal tendon of external oblique aponeurosis
2	Transverse acetabular ligament	6‴	Attachment of pelvic tendon of external oblique aponeurosis on sartorius and iliopsoas ("inguinal ligament")
2′	Femoral head		
3	Pubis		
4	Tunica flava over linea alba	7	Superficial inguinal ring
5	Prepubic tendon	8	Internal abdominal oblique
5′	Accessory ligament	9	Iliopsoas
6	External abdominal oblique	10	Sartorius
6′	Pelvic tendon of external oblique aponeurosis	11	Vascular lacuna containing femoral vessels
		12	Femoral fascia (lamina)

Figure 4-24   Equine abdominal muscles and their skeletal attachments

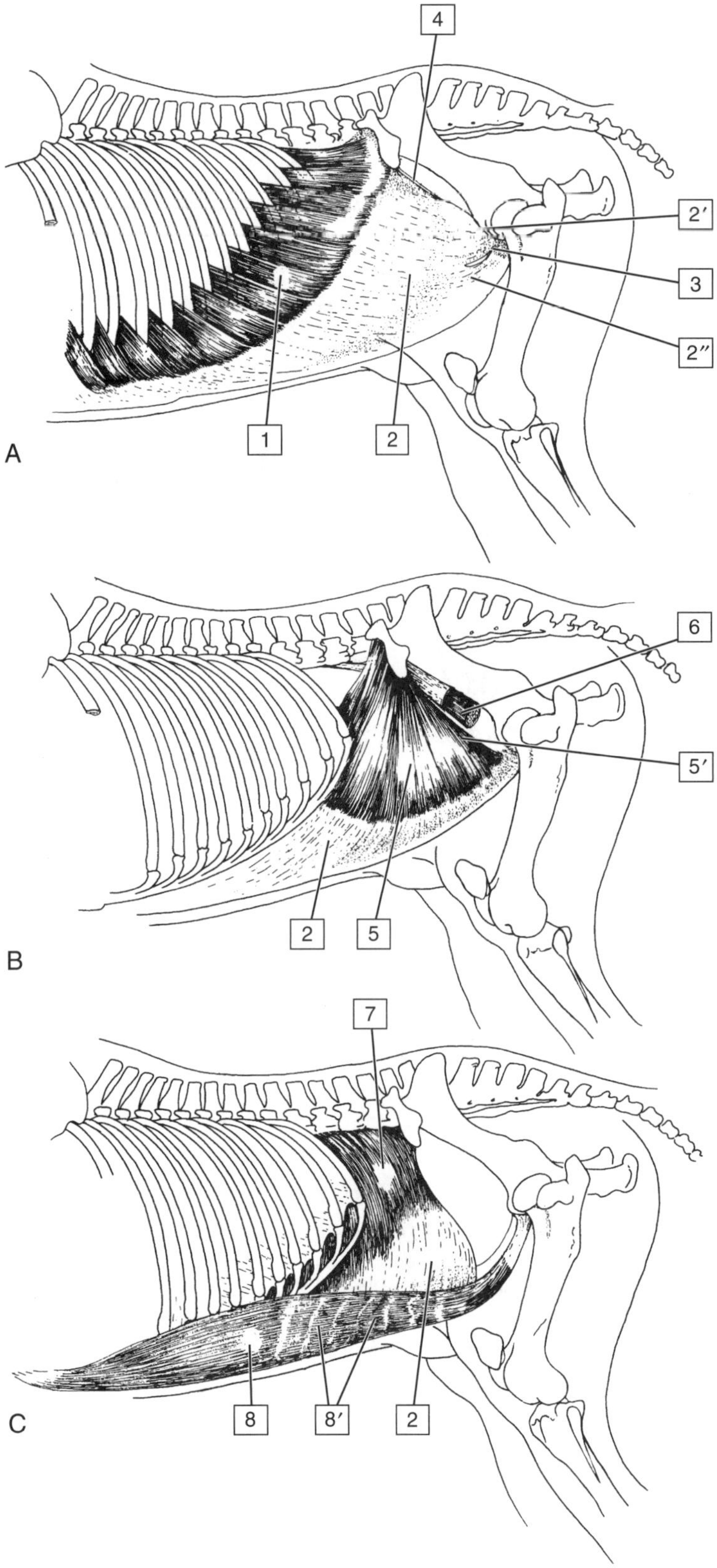

A

B

C

1   External abdominal oblique, muscular part

2   Aponeurotic parts of 1, 5, and 7

2'   Pelvic tendons of aponeurotic part

2"   Abdominal tendons of aponeurotic part

3   Superficial inguinal ring

4   Attachment of pelvic tendon of external oblique aponeurosis on iliopsoas and sartorius ("inguinal ligament")

5   Internal abdominal oblique, muscular part

5'   Free caudal border forming the cranial margin of the deep inguinal ring

6   Iliopsoas, partly enclosed by iliac fascia

7   Transversus abdominis, muscular part

8   Rectus abdominis

8'   Tendinous inscriptions

Figure 4-25   Visceral surface of the equine spleen

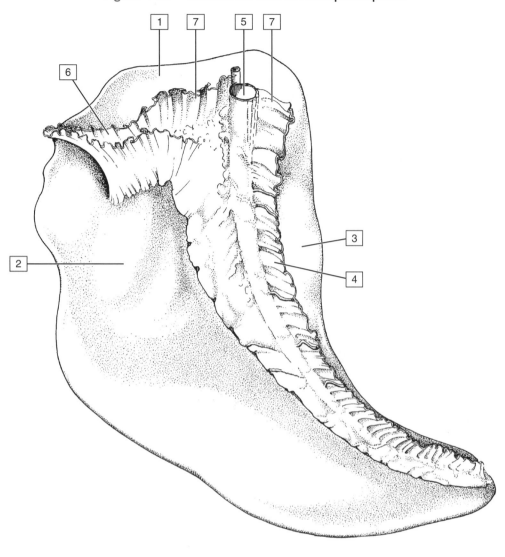

1   Renal surface

2   Intestinal surface

3   Gastric surface

4   Greater omentum (gastrosplenic ligament)

5   Splenic artery and vein

6   Renosplenic ligament

7   Phrenicosplenic ligament

Figure 4-26   Interior of the equine stomach and cranial part of the
duodenum

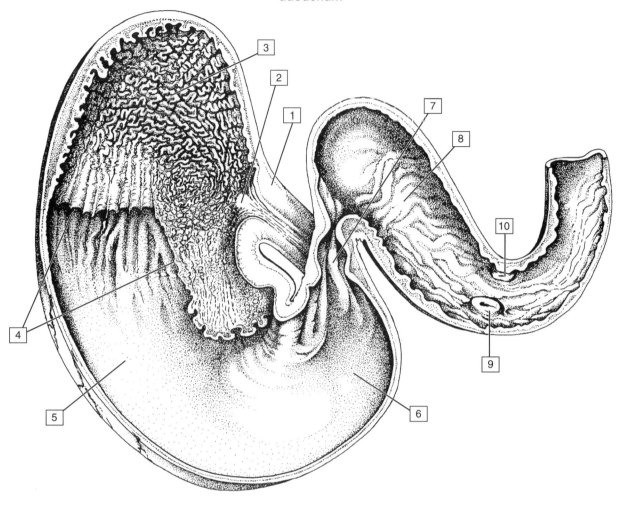

1	Esophagus
2	Cardiac opening
3	Fundus (blind sac)
4	Margo plicatus
5	Body
6	Pyloric part
7	Pylorus
8	Cranial part of duodenum
9	Major duodenal papilla within hepatopancreatic ampulla
10	Minor duodenal papilla

Figure 4-27 Equine intestinal tract seen from the right

The caudal flexure of the duodenum and the cranial mesenteric artery have been displaced to the right of the animal to lie over the base of the cecum.

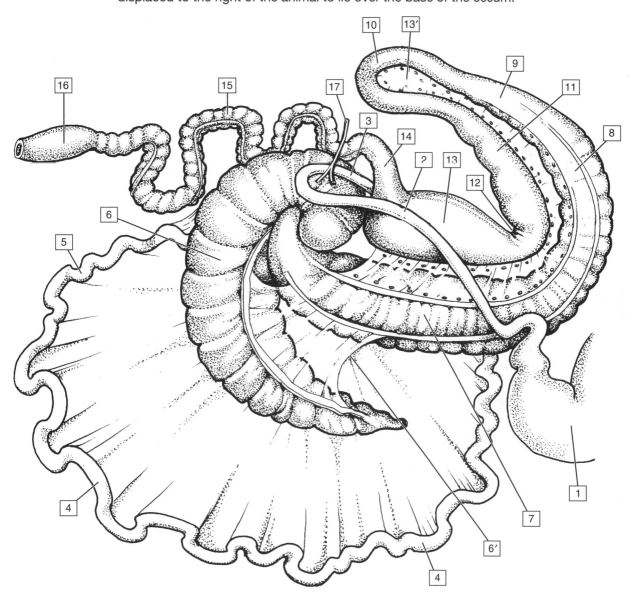

1	Stomach	7	Right ventral colon	13′	Ascending mesocolon
2	Descending duodenum	8	Ventral diaphragmatic flexure	14	Transverse colon
3	Ascending duodenum	9	Left ventral colon	15	Descending (small) colon
4	Jejunum	10	Pelvic flexure	16	Rectum
5	Ileum	11	Left dorsal colon	17	Cranial mesenteric artery
6	Cecum	12	Dorsal diaphragmatic flexure		
6′	Cecocolic fold	13	Right dorsal colon		

Figure 4-28   Position of the equine large intestine and the kidneys, dorsal view

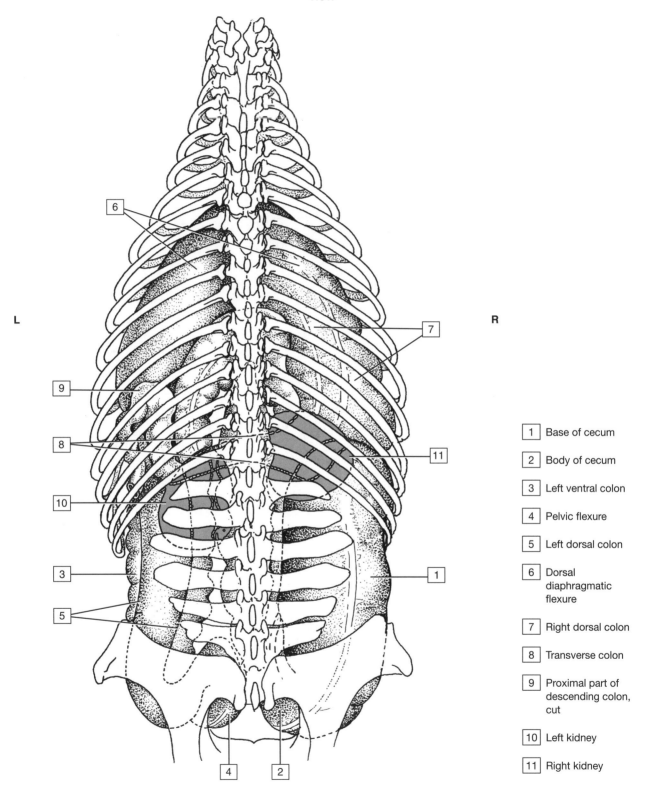

L

R

1	Base of cecum
2	Body of cecum
3	Left ventral colon
4	Pelvic flexure
5	Left dorsal colon
6	Dorsal diaphragmatic flexure
7	Right dorsal colon
8	Transverse colon
9	Proximal part of descending colon, cut
10	Left kidney
11	Right kidney

Figure 4-29   Topography of the equine spleen, stomach, pancreas, and liver, caudoventral view

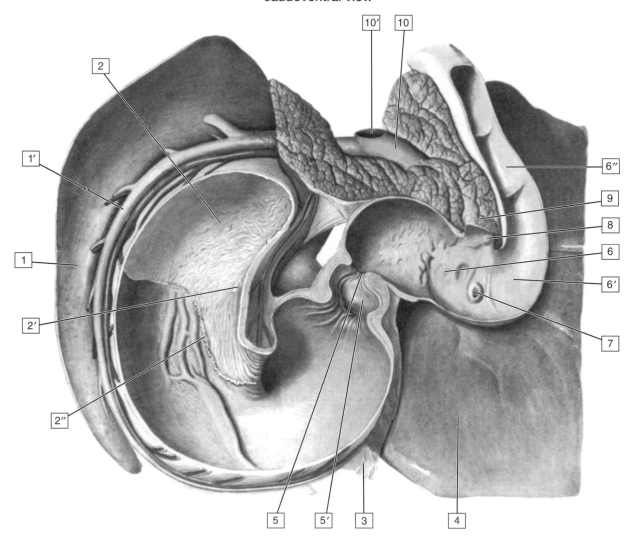

1	Intestinal surface of spleen	6	S-Shaped cranial part of duodenum
1'	Splenic a. and v.	6'	Cranial flexure of duodenum
2	Fundus (blind sac) of stomach	6"	Descending duodenum
2'	Cardia	7	Major duodenal papilla
2"	Margo plicatus	8	Minor duodenal papilla
3	Greater omentum	9	Body of pancreas
4	Liver	10	Portal v.
5	Pyloric orifice	10'	Stump of cranial mesenteric v.
5'	Pyloric antrum		

Figure 4-30   Relationship of the lumbar spinal nerves to the transverse
processes of the bovine lumbar vertebrae

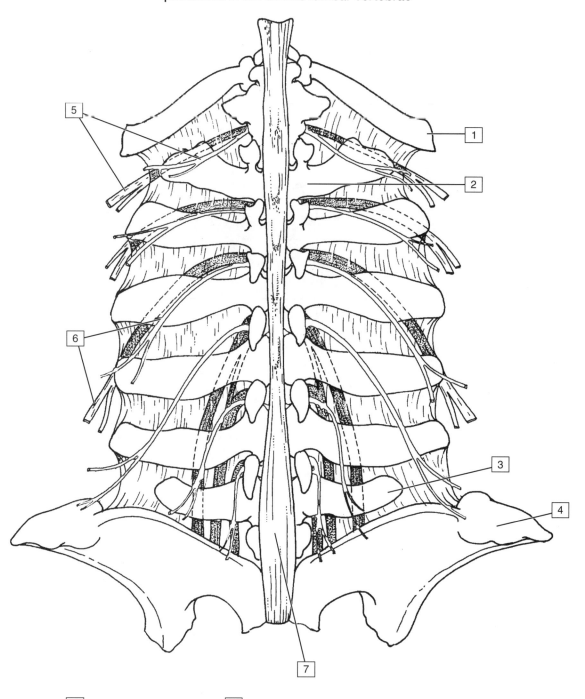

1	Last rib	5	Dorsal and ventral branches of 13th thoracic nerve (the ventral branch is partly stippled)
2	First lumbar vertebra	6	Dorsal and ventral branches of second lumbar nerve
3	Sixth lumbar vertebra	7	Supraspinous ligament
4	Coxal tuber		

Figure 4-31   Topography of the bovine abdominal viscera

A, Relationship of abdominal viscera to the left abdominal wall. *B*, Relationship of abdominal viscera to the right abdominal wall; the liver has been removed.

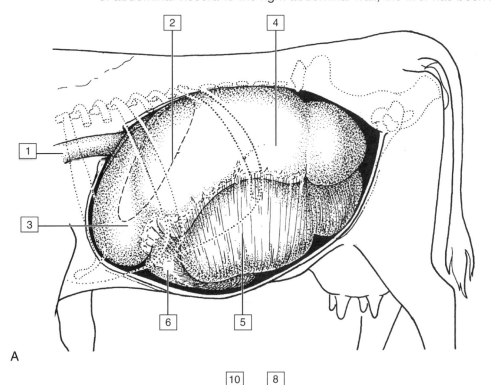

A

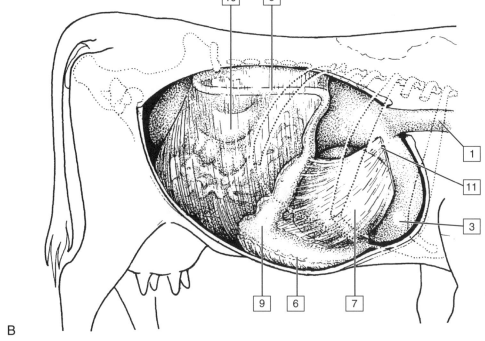

B

1	Esophagus
2	Outline of spleen
3	Reticulum
4	Dorsal sac of rumen
5	Ventral sac of rumen, covered by superficial wall of greater omentum
6	Body of abomasum
7	Omasum, covered by lesser omentum
8	Descending duodenum
9	Pyloric part of abomasum
10	Greater omentum covering the intestinal mass
11	Lesser omentum cut away from the liver

Figure 4-32   Bovine greater omentum fenestrated to permit a view into
omental bursa, caudal view

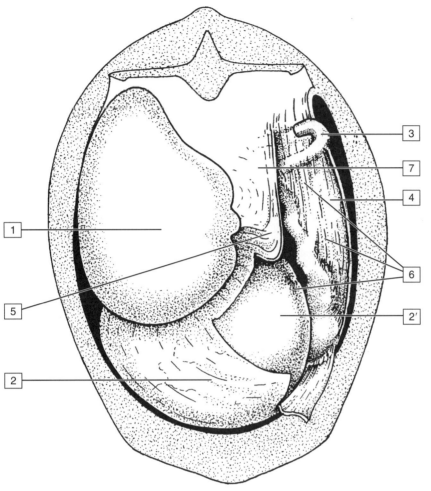

1   Dorsal sac of rumen

2   Ventral sac of rumen, covered
by superficial wall of greater
omentum

2′   Ventral sac of rumen
projecting into omental bursa

3   Caudal flexure of duodenum

4   Superficial wall of greater
omentum

5   Deep wall of greater omentum

6   Omental bursa

7   Supraomental recess

Figure 4-33   Right lateral view of the bovine intestinal tract

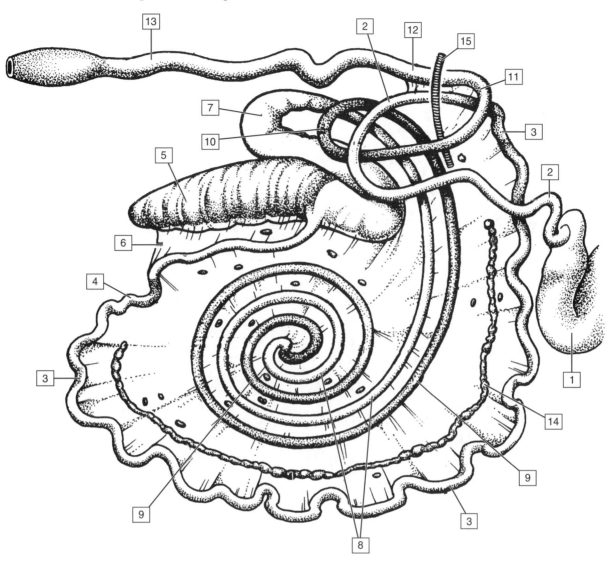

1	Pyloric part of abomasum	8	Centripetal turns of spiral colon
2	Duodenum	9	Centrifugal turns of spiral colon
3	Jejunum	10	Distal loop of ascending colon
4	Ileum	11	Transverse colon
5	Cecum	12	Descending colon
6	Ileocecal fold	13	Rectum

7 to 10, Ascending colon:

7	Proximal loop of ascending colon	14	Jejunal lymph nodes
		15	Cranial mesenteric artery

Figure 4-34   Male porcine inguinal canal, cranial view

Made visible on the interior (deep) surface of the caudal abdominal wall.

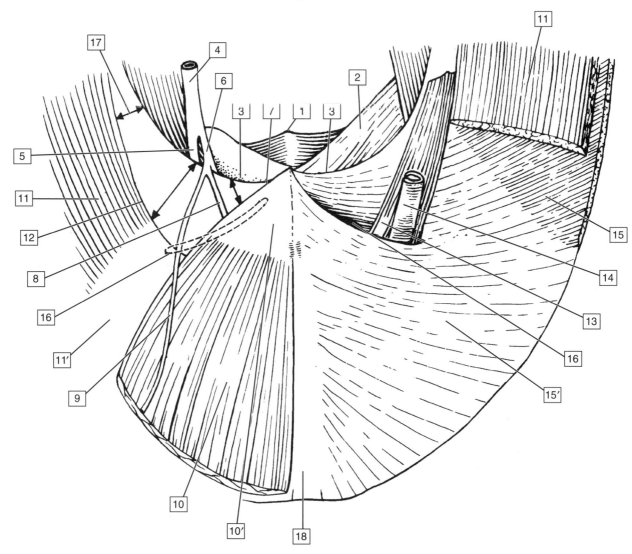

1	Pelvic symphysis	9	Caudal epigastric artery	14	Tunica vaginalis and spermatic cord
2	Prepubic tendon	10	Rectus abdominis	15	Muscular part of external abdominal oblique
3	Caudal border of external oblique aponeurosis ("inguinal ligament")	10'	Rectus tendon	15'	Aponeurotic part of external abdominal oblique
4	External iliac artery	11	Muscular part of internal abdominal oblique	16	Superficial inguinal ring
5	Femoral artery	11'	Aponeurotic part of internal abdominal oblique	17	Deep inguinal ring *(arrows)*
6	Deep femoral artery	12	Caudal free border of internal abdominal oblique	18	Linea alba
7	Lateral border of rectus tendon	13	Cremaster		
8	External pudendal artery				

Figure 4-35 Development of the porcine ascending colon, left lateral view

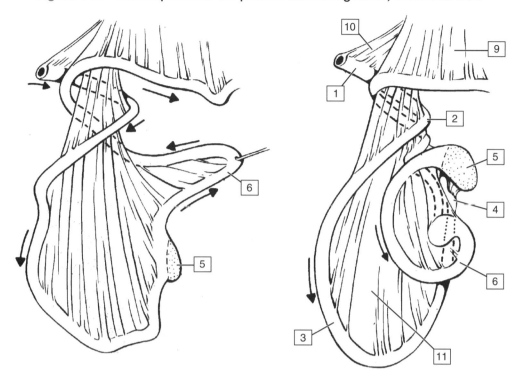

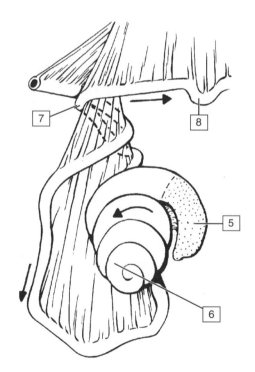

1	Descending duodenum	5	Cecum	9	Descending mesocolon
2	Caudal flexure of duodenum	6	Ascending colon	10	Mesoduodenum
3	Jejunum	7	Transverse colon	11	Mesentery
4	Ileum	8	Descending colon		

Figure 4-36   Major porcine abdominal arteries and lymph nodes

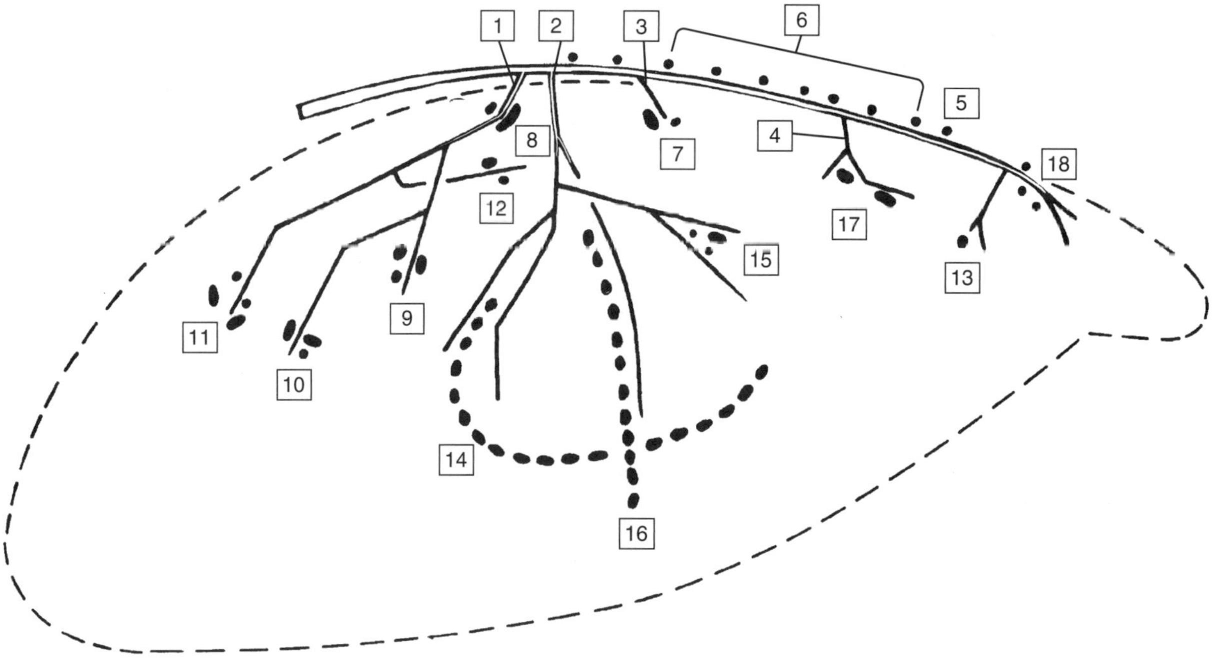

1	Celiac artery	10	Gastric nodes
2	Cranial mesenteric artery	11	Hepatic nodes
3	Renal artery	12	Pancreaticoduodenal nodes
4	Caudal mesenteric artery	13	Lateral iliac nodes
5	Deep circumflex iliac artery	14	Jejunal nodes
6	Lumbar aortic nodes	15	Ileocolic nodes
7	Renal nodes	16	Colic nodes
8	Celiac nodes	17	Caudal mesenteric nodes
9	Splenic nodes	18	Medial iliac nodes

Figure 4-37   Avian gastrointestinal tract after reflection of liver, stomach, and small intestine craniodextrally, ventral view

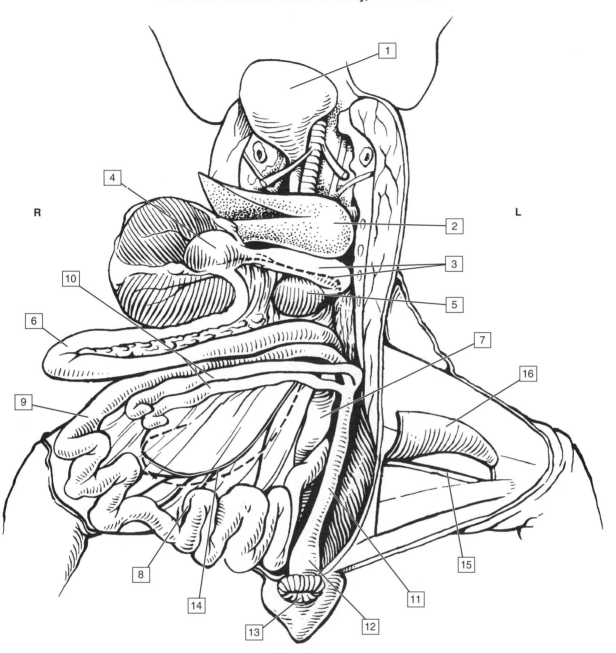

1 Crop	6 Duodenal loop enclosing pancreas	12 Cloaca
2 Left lobe of liver	7 Jejunum	13 Vent
3 Proventriculus with vagus on dorsal surface	8 Vitelline diverticulum	14 Cranial mesenteric vessels and intestinal nerve in mesentery
4 Cranial blind sac on right side of reflected gizzard	9 Ileum	15 Sciatic nerve and ischial artery
5 Spleen	10 Ceca	16 Gracilis and adductor
	11 Colon	

Figure 4-38   Canine, equine, and bovine gastrointestinal tracts laid out in one plane

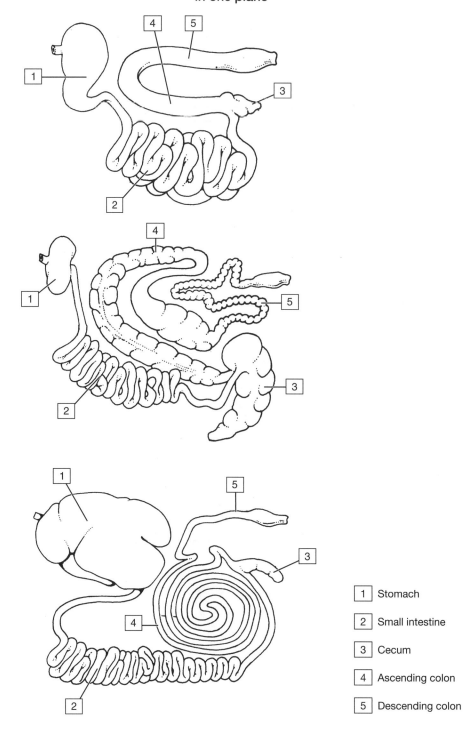

1	Stomach
2	Small intestine
3	Cecum
4	Ascending colon
5	Descending colon

Figure 4-39   Canine and feline (*A*), porcine (*B*), bovine (*C*), and equine (*D*) large intestine

Cranial is to the upper right.

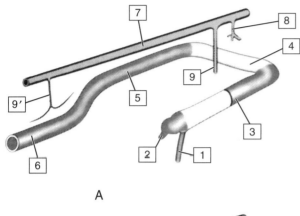

A

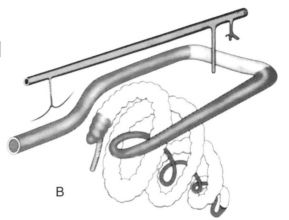

B

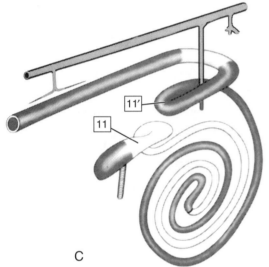

C

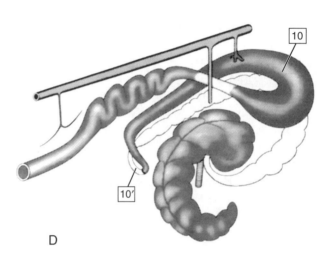

D

1	Ileum	8	Celiac artery
2	Cecum	9	Cranial mesenteric artery
3	Ascending colon	9′	Caudal mesenteric artery
4	Transverse colon	10	Dorsal diaphragmatic flexures of ascending colon
5	Descending colon	10′	Pelvic flexures of ascending colon
6	Rectum and anus	11	Proximal loop of ascending colon
7	Aorta	11′	Distal loop of ascending colon

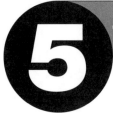

THE PELVIS AND REPRODUCTIVE ORGANS

Figure 5-1   Canine sacrum, cranial view

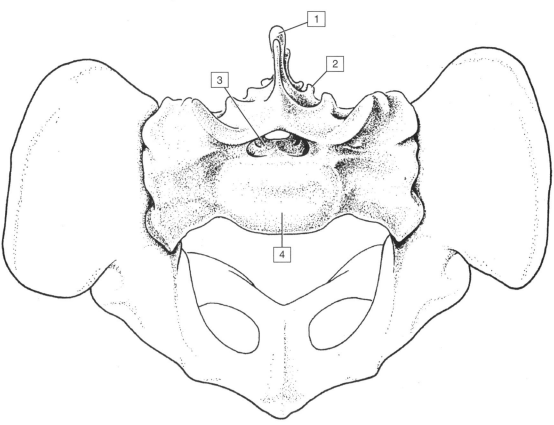

1	Spinous process
2	Rudimentary articular process
3	Vertebral canal
4	Body

Figure 5-2   Sagittal section of an early canine embryo

Part of the yolk sac is taken into the body in the folding process.

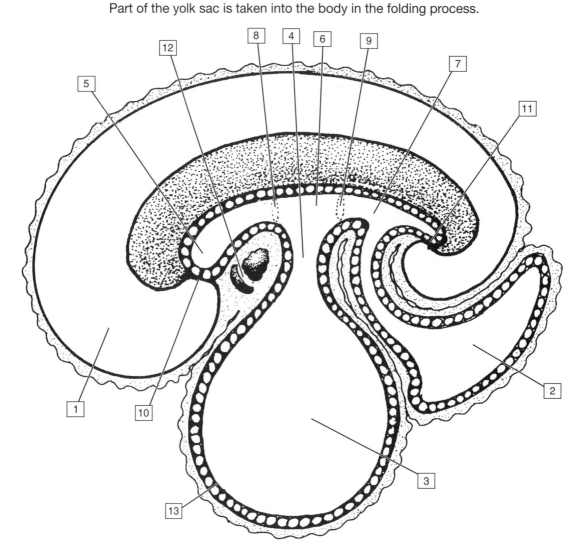

1 Amniotic cavity	8 Cranial intestinal portal
2 Allantoic cavity	9 Caudal intestinal portal
3 Yolk sac	10 Oral plate
4 Stalk of yolk sac	11 Cloacal plate
5 Foregut	12 Heart and pericardial cavity
6 Midgut	13 Endoderm
7 Hindgut	

Figure 5-3   Canine urinary and male and female reproductive organs

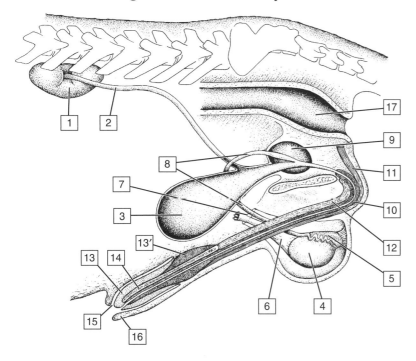

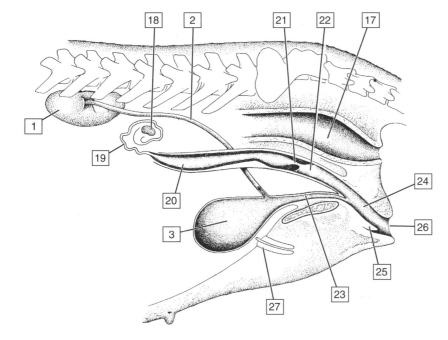

1	Right kidney
2	Ureter
3	Bladder
4	Testis
5	Epididymis
6	Spermatic cord
7	Vaginal ring
8	Deferent duct
9	Prostate
10	Corpus spongiosum (spongy body)
11	Retractor penis
12	Corpus cavernosum (cavernous body)
13	Glans penis
13'	Bulb of glans
14	Os penis
15	Preputial cavity
16	Prepuce
17	Rectum
18	Ovary
19	Uterine tube
20	Uterine horn
21	Cervix
22	Vagina
23	Urethra
24	Vestibule
25	Clitoris
26	Vulva
27	Vaginal process

Figure 5-4 Three stages in the development of the canine testis

A, The epithelial cords are isolated from the surface epithelium by the formation of the tunica albuginea. *B*, The epithelial cords, rete, and mesonephric tubules have interconnected. *C*, The epithelial cords become seminiferous tubules, and the mesonephros is gradually transformed into part of the epididymis.

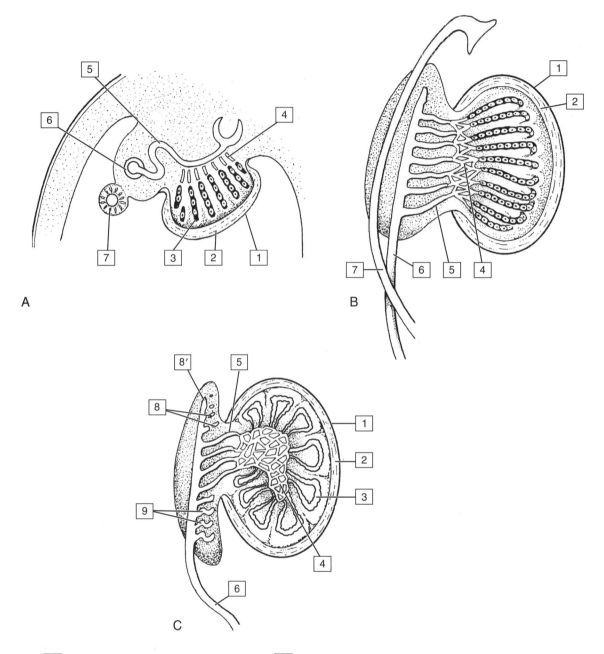

1	Celom epithelium	6	Mesonephric (later deferent) duct
2	Tunica albuginea	7	Paramesonephric duct
3	Epithelial cords, seminiferous tubules	8	Cranial remnant of mesonephric tubules (aberrant ductules)
4	Rete testis	8'	Remnant of 6 (appendix of epididymis)
5	Mesonephric tubules, efferent ductules	9	Caudal remnant (paradidymis)

Figure 5-5   Canine kidney lobe

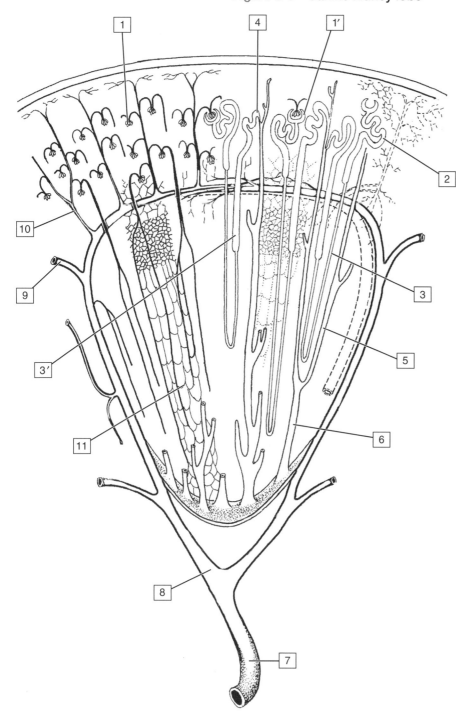

1	Glomerulus
1′	Renal corpuscle
2	Proximal convoluted tubule
3	Descending limb of nephron
3′	Ascending limb
4	Distal convoluted tubule
5	Collecting tubule
6	Papillary duct
7	Renal artery
8	Interlobar artery
9	Arcuate artery
10	Interlobular artery
11	Capillary plexus

Figure 5-6   Longitudinal section of canine testis and epididymis

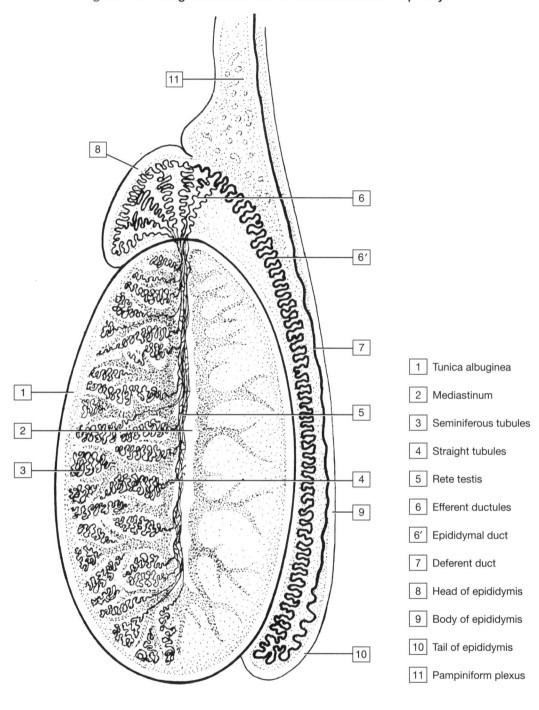

1	Tunica albuginea
2	Mediastinum
3	Seminiferous tubules
4	Straight tubules
5	Rete testis
6	Efferent ductules
6′	Epididymal duct
7	Deferent duct
8	Head of epididymis
9	Body of epididymis
10	Tail of epididymis
11	Pampiniform plexus

Figure 5-7   Different functional stages in canine ovarian activity

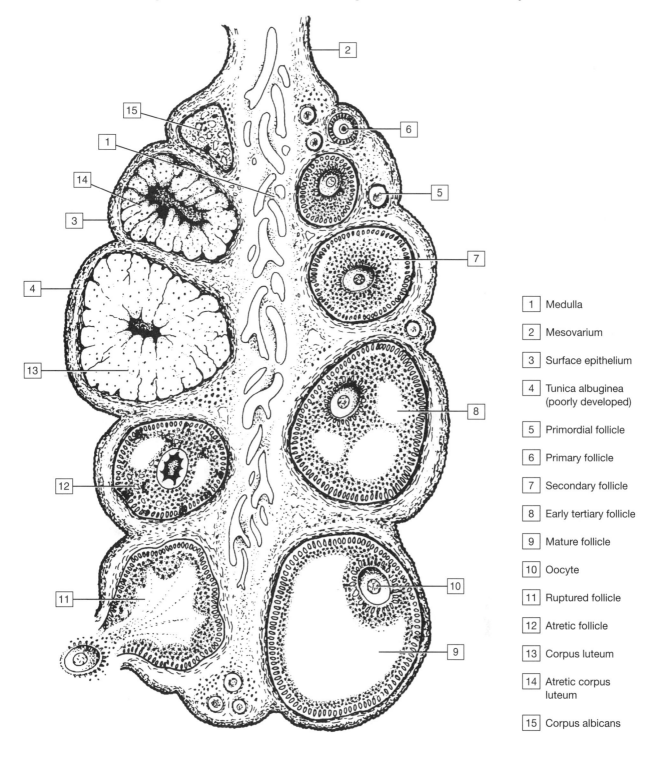

1	Medulla
2	Mesovarium
3	Surface epithelium
4	Tunica albuginea (poorly developed)
5	Primordial follicle
6	Primary follicle
7	Secondary follicle
8	Early tertiary follicle
9	Mature follicle
10	Oocyte
11	Ruptured follicle
12	Atretic follicle
13	Corpus luteum
14	Atretic corpus luteum
15	Corpus albicans

Figure 5-8   Blood supply of the female canine reproductive tract

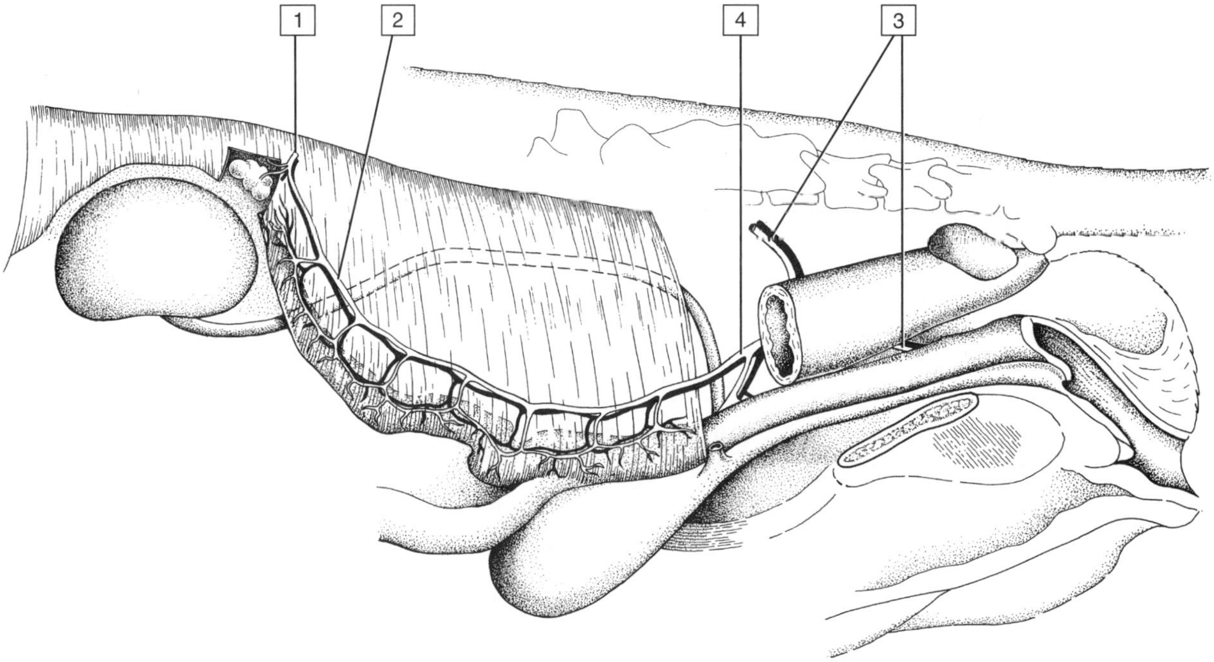

1	Ovarian artery
2	Uterine branch of the ovarian artery
3	Vaginal artery
4	Uterine artery

Figure 5-9   Formation of canine extraembryonic membranes

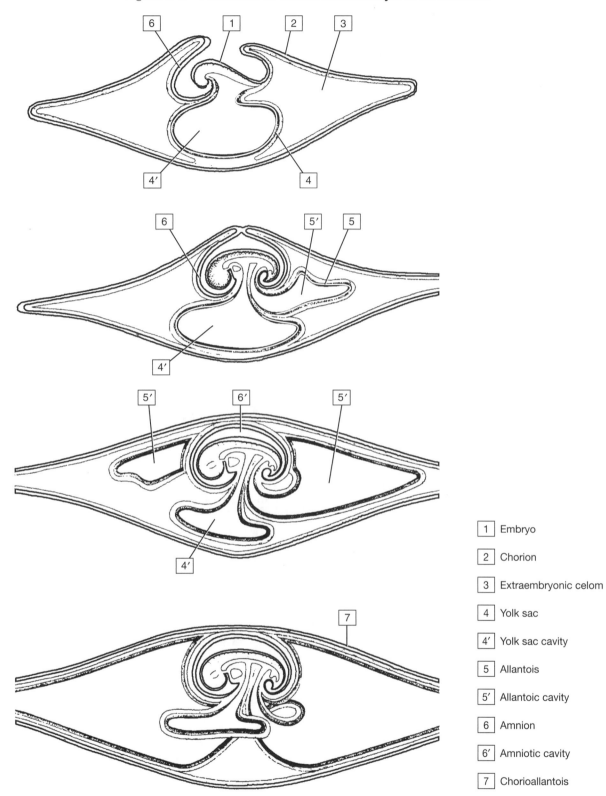

1 Embryo

2 Chorion

3 Extraembryonic celom

4 Yolk sac

4′ Yolk sac cavity

5 Allantois

5′ Allantoic cavity

6 Amnion

6′ Amniotic cavity

7 Chorioallantois

Figure 5-10   Transverse section of the canine pelvis at the level of the hip
joint

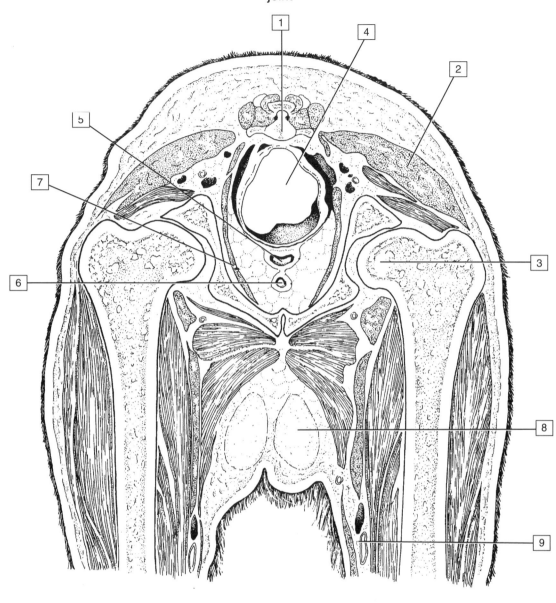

1	Caudal vertebra	6	Urethra
2	Superficial gluteal muscle	7	Levator ani
3	Head of femur in acetabulum	8	Inguinal mammary gland
4	Rectum suspended by a short mesorectum	9	Femoral artery and vein
5	Vagina		

Figure 5-11   Deep dissection of the external canine reproductive organs

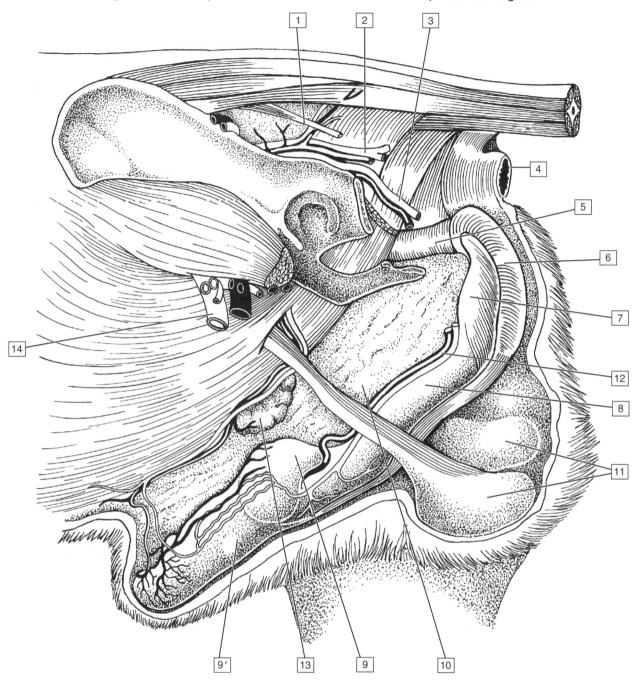

1	Sacrotuberous ligament
2	Caudal gluteal vessels
3	Internal pudendal vessels
4	Anus
5	Pelvic urethra
6	Bulb of penis enclosed by bulbospongiosus
7	Ischiocavernosus over left cms
8	Body of penis
9	Bulbus glandis
9′	Pars longa glandis
10	Spermatic cord
11	Testes in scrotum
12	Dorsal artery and vein of the penis
13	Superficial inguinal lymph nodes and caudal superficial epigastric vessels
14	Femoral vessels

Figure 5-12   Right canine lumbosacral nerves and left arteries, ventral view

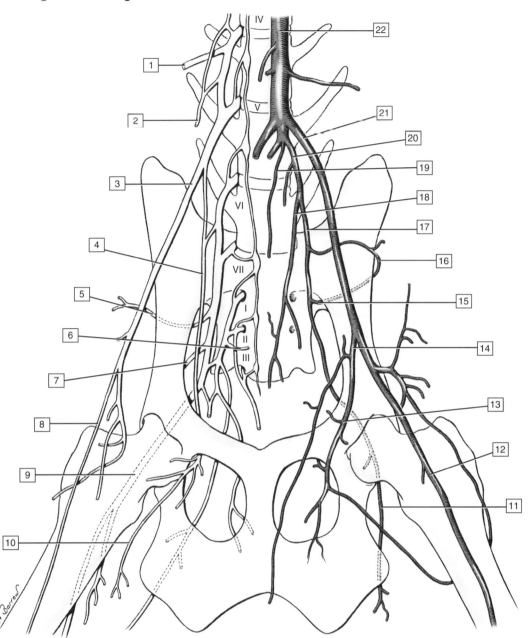

1	Lateral cutaneous femoral nerve	7	Caudal gluteal nerve	13	Medial circumflex femoral artery	19	Median sacral artery
2	Genitofemoral nerve	8	Saphenous nerve	14	Deep femoral artery	20	Internal iliac artery
3	Femoral nerve	9	Sciatic nerve	15	Cranial gluteal artery	21	External iliac artery
4	Obturator nerve	10	Obturator nerve	16	Iliolumbar artery	22	Aorta
5	Cranial gluteal nerve	11	Caudal gluteal nerve	17	Caudal gluteal artery		
6	Pelvic nerve	12	Femoral artery	18	Internal pudendal artery		

Figure 5-13   Canine nerves, arteries, and muscles of the right hip, lateral aspect

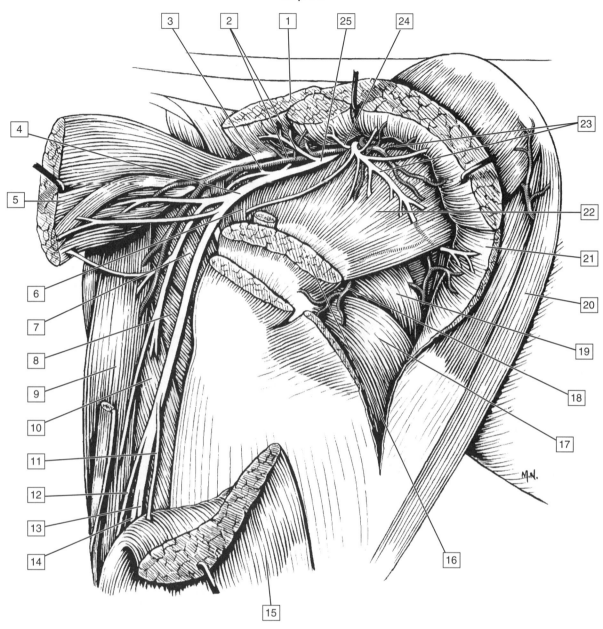

1 Superficial gluteus	7 Quadratus femoris	14 Tibial nerve	21 Tensor fasciae latae
2 Caudal gluteal artery and nerve	8 Adductor	15 Biceps femoris	22 Deep gluteal
3 Nerve to internal obturator, gemelli, and quadratus femoris	9 Semitendinosus	16 Middle gluteal	23 Cranial gluteal artery and nerve
	10 Semimembranosus	17 Vastus lateralis	24 Nerve to piriformis
4 Sciatic nerve	11 Lateral cutaneous sural nerve	18 Lateral circumflex femoral artery	25 Lumbosacral trunk
5 Biceps femoris	12 Caudal cutaneous sural nerve	19 Rectus femoris	
6 Gemelli	13 Common fibular nerve	20 Sartorius	

Figure 5-14   The reproductive organs of the tomcat in situ, left lateral view

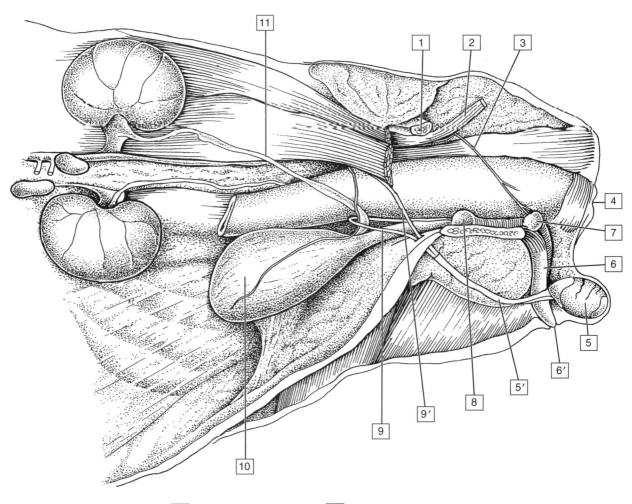

1	Shaft of ilium	6′	Prepuce
2	Sciatic nerve	7	Bulbourethral gland
3	Pudendal nerve	8	Prostate
4	Anus	9	Deferent duct
5	Left testis in scrotum	9′	Testicular vessels
5′	Spermatic cord	10	Bladder
6	Penis	11	Left ureter

Saunders Veterinary Anatomy Coloring Book
Copyright © 2011 by Saunders, an imprint of Elsevier Inc.

Figure 5-15   Median section of the pelvis of the mare and caudal abdominal and pelvic organs of the mare in situ

The organs have been sectioned in a paramedian plane with the pelvis. Because of the absence of the intestines, the ovaries hang much lower than they would in the intact animal.

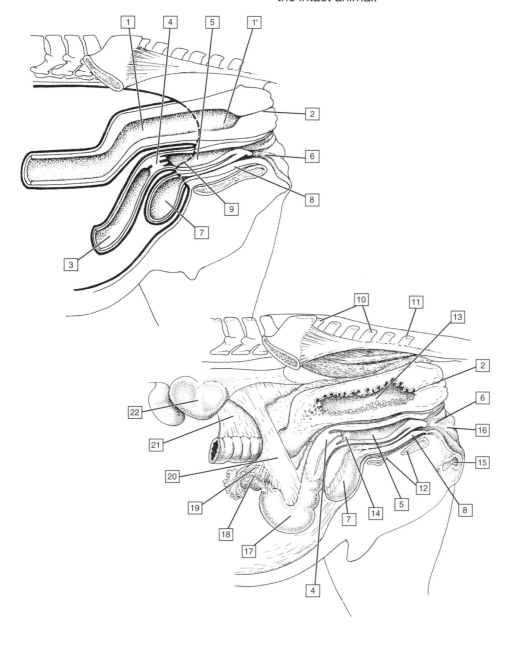

1	Peritoneal part of the rectum
1'	Retroperitoneal parts of the rectum
2	Anal canal
3	Uterus
4	Cervix
5	Vagina
6	Vestibule
7	Bladder
8	Urethra
9	Caudal extent of peritoneum
10	Sacrum
11	Cd2
12	Floor of pelvis
13	Rectum
14	Vaginal part of cervix
15	Clitoris
16	Vulva
17	Left uterine horn
18	Uterine tube
19	Ovary
20	Broad ligament (largely cut away)
21	Descending mesocolon
22	Left kidney

Figure 5-16 Equine right ovary, uterine tube, and uterine horn, lateral view

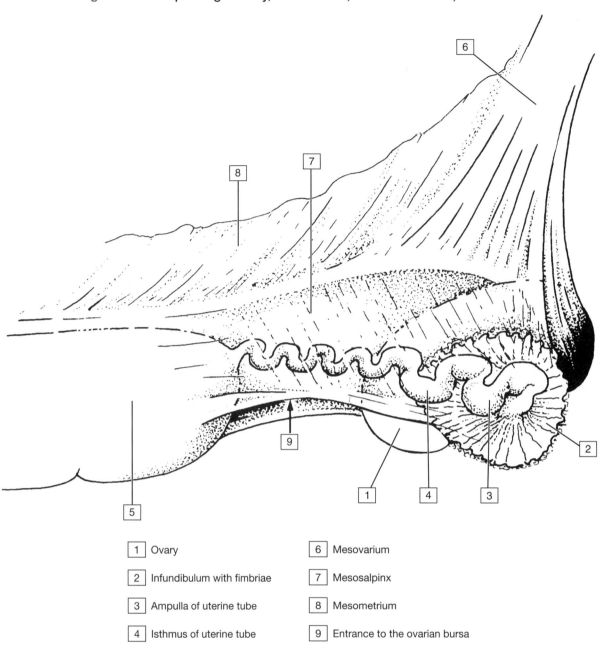

1	Ovary	6	Mesovarium
2	Infundibulum with fimbriae	7	Mesosalpinx
3	Ampulla of uterine tube	8	Mesometrium
4	Isthmus of uterine tube	9	Entrance to the ovarian bursa
5	Uterine horn		

Figure 5-17   Branching pattern of the caudal part of the bovine abdominal aorta

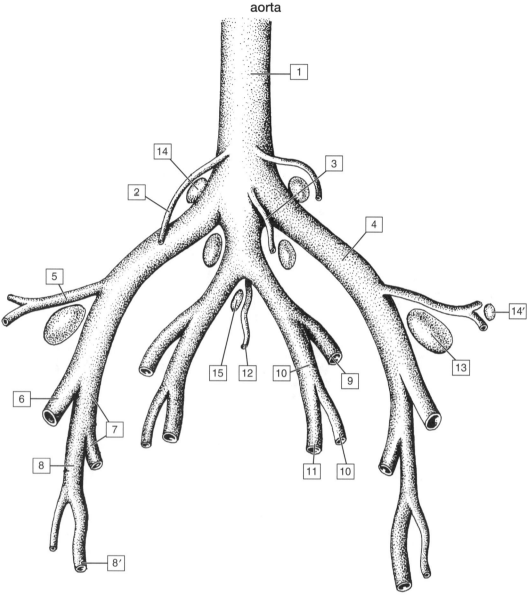

1 Aorta	9 Internal iliac artery
2 Ovarian artery	10 Umbilical artery
3 Caudal mesenteric artery	11 Uterine artery
4 External iliac artery	12 Median sacral artery
5 Deep circumflex iliac artery	13 Deep inguinal (iliofemoral) lymph node
6 Femoral artery	14 Medial iliac lymph node
7 Deep femoral artery	14′ Lateral iliac lymph nodes
8 Pudendoepigastric trunk	15 Sacral lymph nodes
8′ External pudendal artery	

Figure 5-18 Nerves and vessels on the medial surface of the bovine pelvic wall

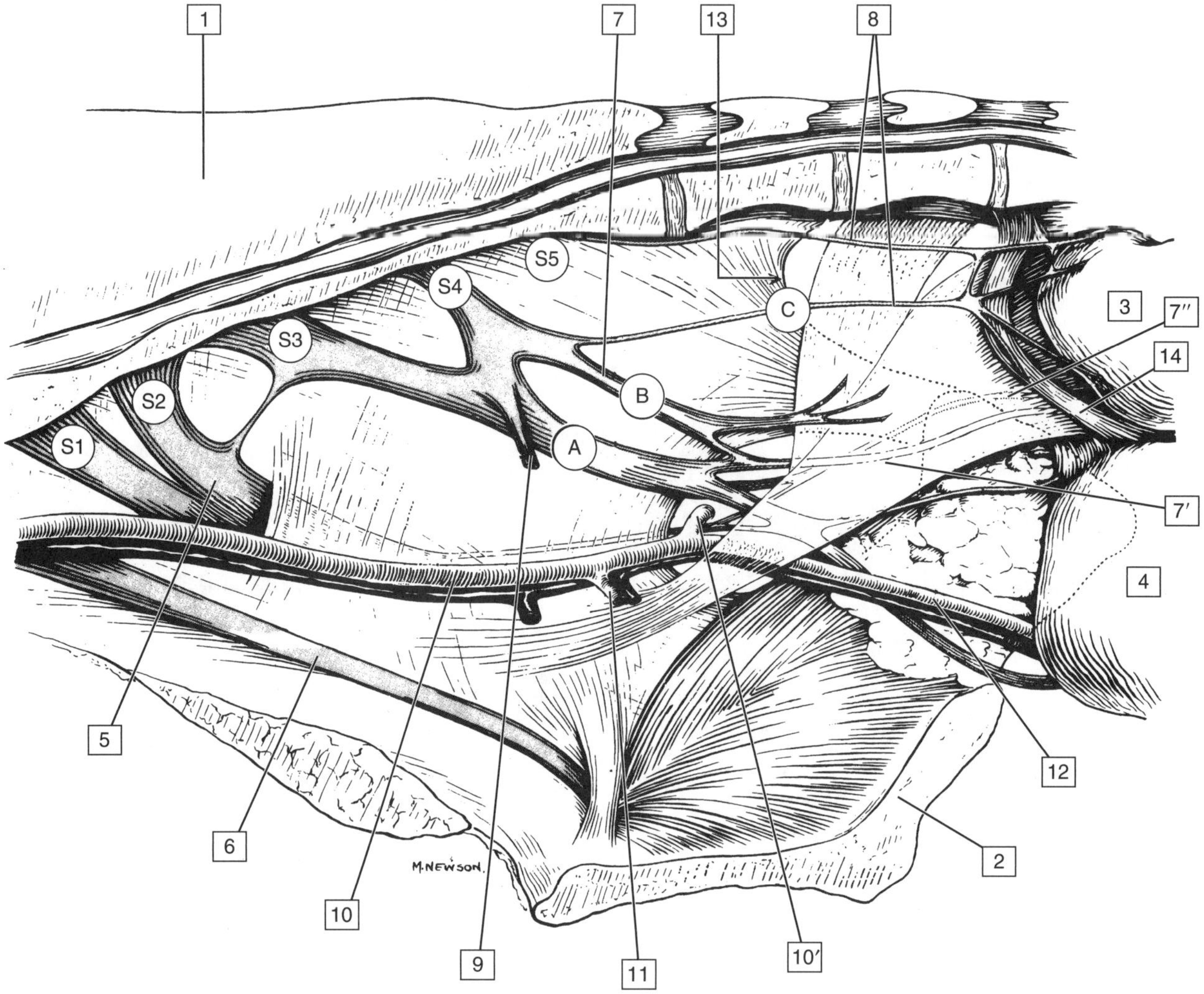

Local anesthesia of the pudendal nerve can be obtained by injections at A and B. Anesthesia of the caudal rectal nerves is possible by injection at C.

1	Sacrum	7	Pudendal n.	10	Internal iliac a.
2	Pelvic symphysis	7′	Distal cutaneous branch of pudendal n.	10′	Caudal gluteal a.
3	Rectum (reflected)	7″	Proximal cutaneous branch of pudendal n.	11	Vaginal a.
4	Vagina (reflected)	8	Caudal rectal n.	12	Internal pudendal a.
5	Sciatic n.	9	Pelvic n.	13	Caudal border of sacrosciatic ligament
6	Obturator n.			14	Retractor clitoridis

Figure 5-19   The bovine reproductive organs, dorsal view

The uterus, cervix, vagina, and vestibule have been opened.

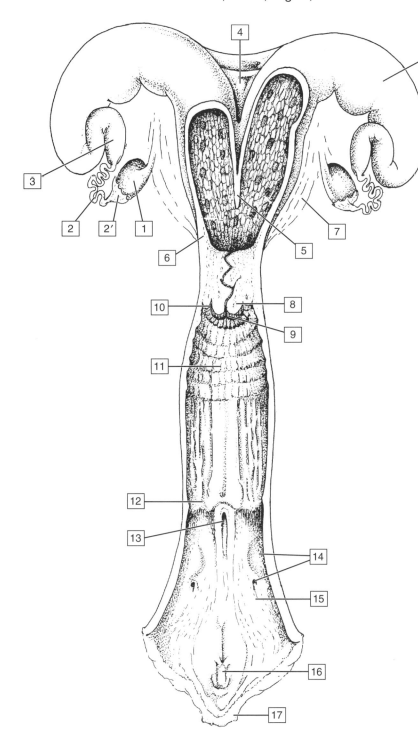

1	Ovary
2	Uterine tube
2'	Infundibulum
3	Uterine horn
4	Intercornual ligament
5	Wall of uterus dividing the two horns
6	Body of uterus with caruncles
7	Broad ligament
8	Cervix
9	Vaginal part of cervix
10	Fornix
11	Vagina
12	Position of former hymen
13	External urethral orifice and suburethral diverticulum
14	Major vestibular gland and its excretory orifice
15	Vestibule
16	Glans of the clitoris
17	Right labium

Figure 5-20   The bovine penis and its muscles, caudolateral view

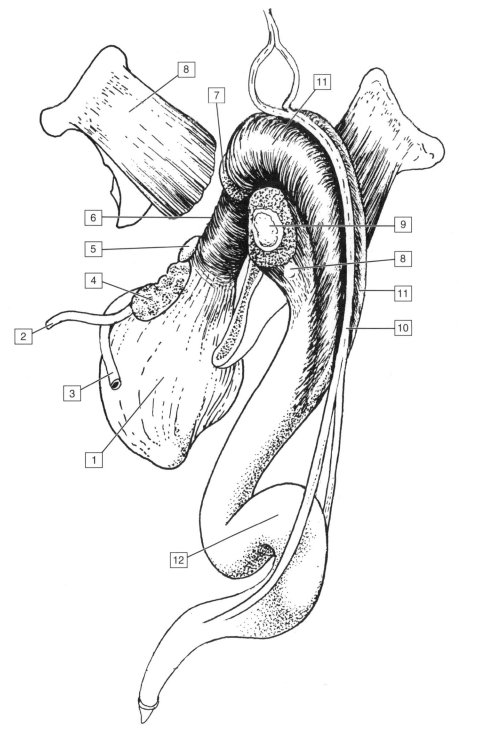

1	Bladder
2	Ureter
3	Deferent duct
4	Vesicular gland
5	Body of prostate
6	Urethralis
7	Bulbourethral gland
8	Ischiocavernosus
9	Crus of penis (in tranverse section)
10	Retractor penis
11	Bulbospongiosus
12	Sigmoid flexure

Figure 5-21   Bovine venous and lymph drainage of the udder

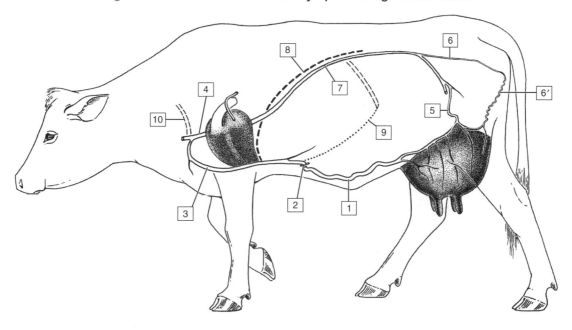

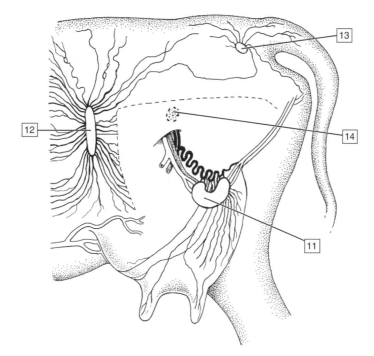

1	Subcutaneous abdominal (milk) v.	6	Internal pudendal v.	10	First rib
2	Milk "well"	6'	Ventral labial v. (connecting ventral perineal v. with caudal mammary veins)	11	Mammary (superficial inguinal) lymph node
3	Internal thoracic v.	7	Caudal vena cava	12	Subiliac lymph node
4	Cranial vena cava	8	Diaphragm	13	Ischial lymph node
5	External pudendal v.	9	Costal arch	14	Position of deep inguinal (iliofemoral) node

Figure 5-22   Cranial view of the opened scrotum of a bull

The investments of the testis have been partly dissected.

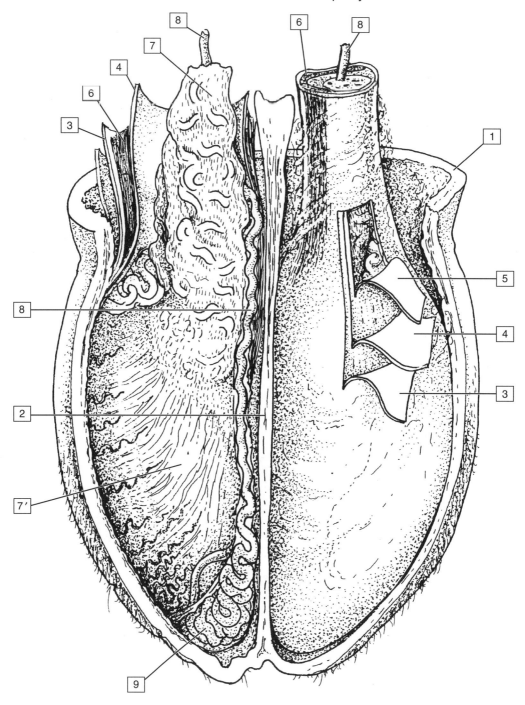

1 Scrotal skin and dartos	5 Visceral layer (dissected from surface of testis)	7′ Visceral layer on testis
2 Scrotal septum	6 Cremaster muscle	8 Deferent duct
3 External spermatic fascia	7 Visceral layer of vaginal tunic covering structures in spermatic cord	9 Tail of epididymis
4 Parietal layer of vaginal tunic		

Figure 5-23   Ventral and lateral views of the abdominal roof in a pig embryo
of 2.5 cm

The pronephric duct drains the mesonephros and is now more aptly termed the
mesonephric duct.

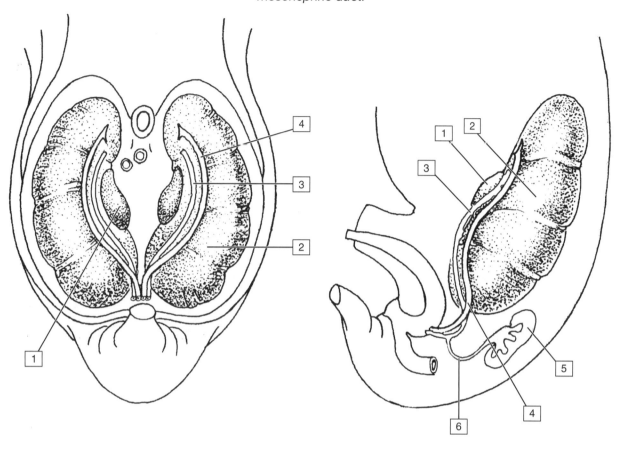

1	Developing gonad
2	Mesonephros
3	Mesonephric duct
4	Paramesonephric duct
5	Metanephros
6	Ureter

Figure 5-24   The development of the metanephrons from two primordia
(metanephric cord and ureteric bud)

Note the gradual regression of the mesonephros.

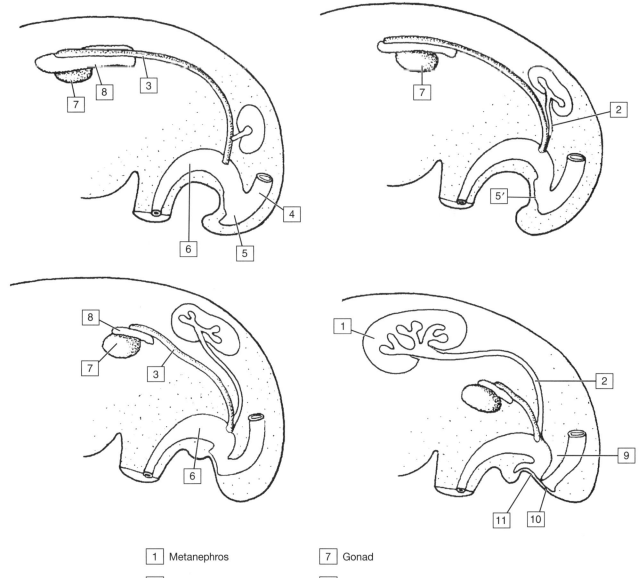

1	Metanephros	7	Gonad
2	Ureteric bud (future ureter)	8	Remnant of mesonephros (future epididymis)
3	Mesonephric (deferent) duct	9	Urorectal septum
4	Rectum	10	Anal membrane
5	Cloaca	11	Urogenital membrane
5′	Cloacal membrane		
6	Urogenital sinus		

Saunders Veterinary Anatomy Coloring Book
Copyright © 2011 by Saunders, an imprint of Elsevier Inc.

Figure 5-25   Transverse section of the free end of the porcine penis

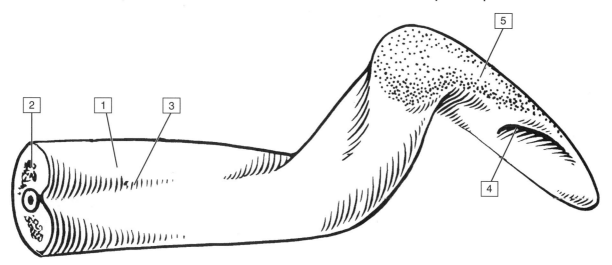

1	Tunica albuginea
2	Corpus cavernosum
3	Urethral groove
4	External urethral orifice
5	Thin glans penis

Figure 6-1   Canine left humerus, cranial view

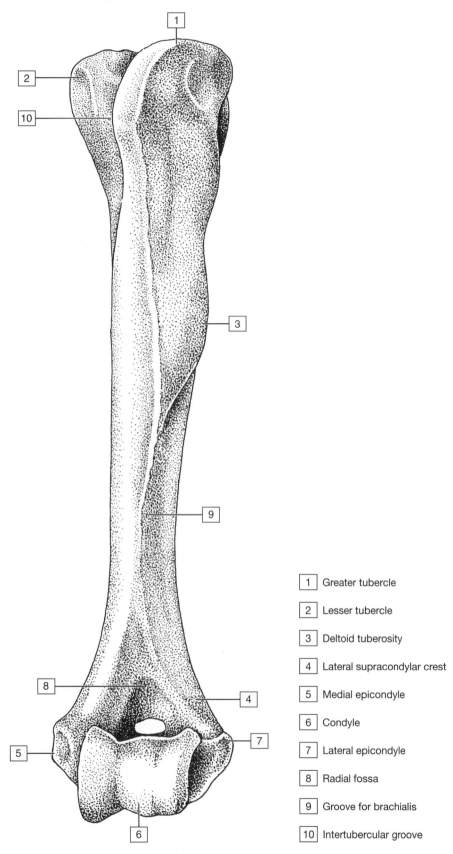

1   Greater tubercle

2   Lesser tubercle

3   Deltoid tuberosity

4   Lateral supracondylar crest

5   Medial epicondyle

6   Condyle

7   Lateral epicondyle

8   Radial fossa

9   Groove for brachialis

10 Intertubercular groove

Figure 6-2   Canine left ulna and left radius

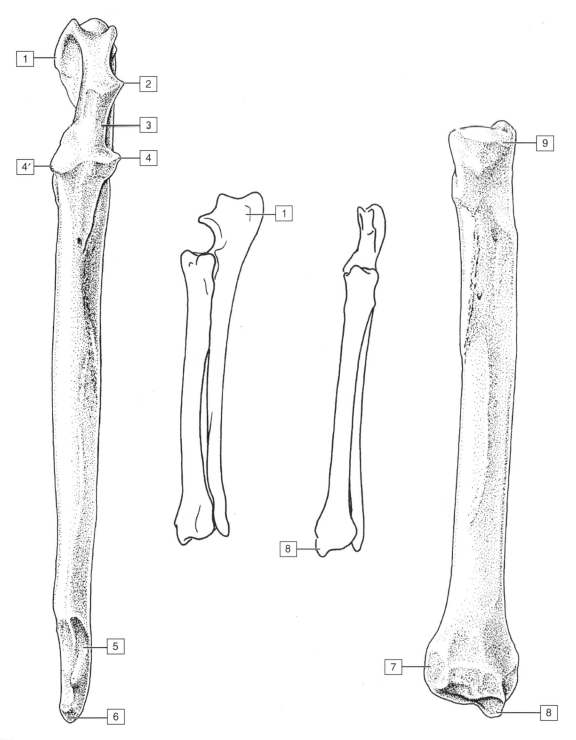

1 Olecranon	4′ Medial coronoid process	7 Articular facet for ulna
2 Anconeal process	5 Distal articular facet for radius	8 Medial styloid process
3 Trochlear notch	6 Lateral styloid process (with facet for the ulnar carpal bone in the dog)	9 Circumferential facet
4 Lateral coronoid process		

Saunders Veterinary Anatomy Coloring Book
Copyright © 2011 by Saunders, an imprint of Elsevier Inc.

Figure 6-3 Superficial muscles of the canine shoulder and arm

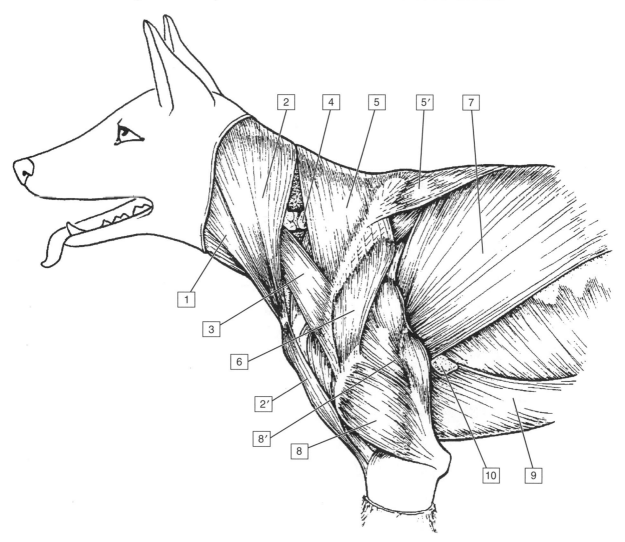

1	Sternocephalicus	6	Deltoideus
2	Brachiocephalicus: cleidocervicalis and cleidobrachialis	7	Latissimus dorsi
2′	Brachiocephalicus: cleidocervicalis and cleidobrachialis	8	Lateral head of triceps
3	Omotransversarius	8′	Long head of triceps
4	Superficial cervical lymph node	9	Pectoralis profundus (ascendens)
5	Cervical part of trapezius	10	Accessory axillary lymph node
5′	Thoracic part of trapezius		

Figure 6-4   Intrinsic muscles of the canine left shoulder and arm, lateral and medial views

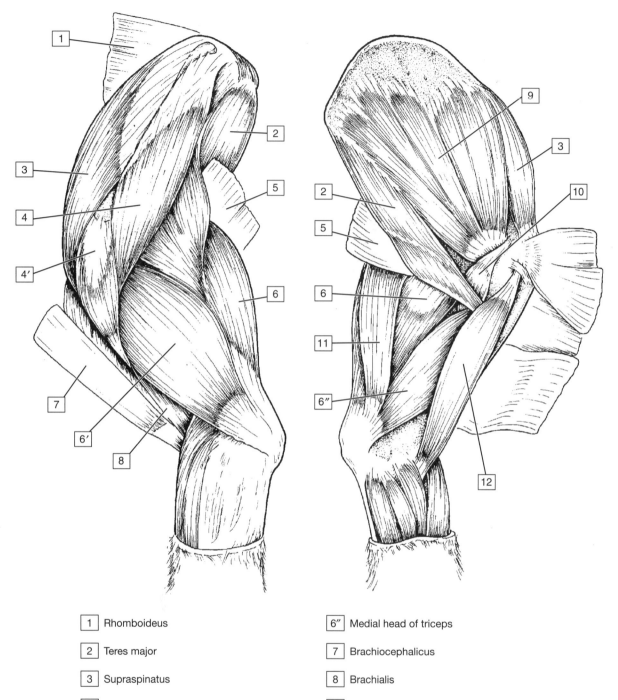

1 Rhomboideus	6″ Medial head of triceps
2 Teres major	7 Brachiocephalicus
3 Supraspinatus	8 Brachialis
4 Scapular part of deltoideus	9 Subscapularis
4′ Acromial part of deltoideus	10 Coracobrachialis
5 Latissimus dorsi	11 Tensor fasciae antebrachii
6 Long, head of triceps	12 Biceps
6′ Lateral head of triceps	

Figure 6-5   Muscles of the canine left forearm, lateral and medial views

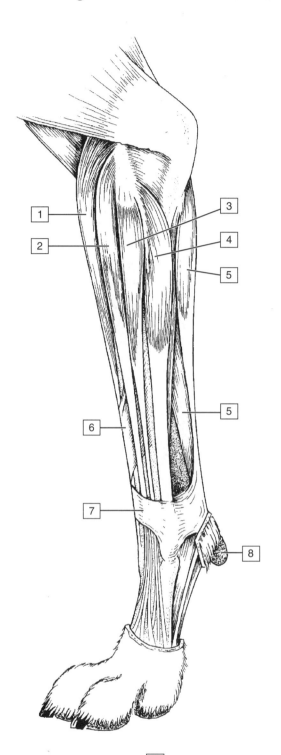

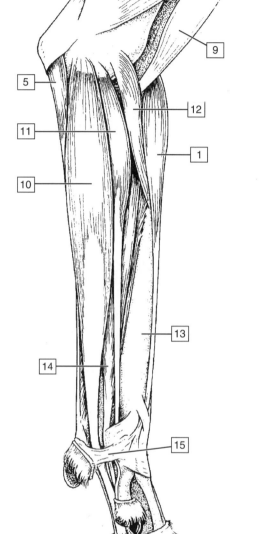

1	Extensor carpi radialis	5	Flexor carpi ulnaris
2	Common digital extensor	6	Extensor carpi obliquus
3	Lateral digital extensor	7	Extensor retinaculum
4	Ulnaris lateralis	8	Carpal pad

9	Biceps	13	Radius
10	Superficial digital flexor	14	Deep digital flexor
11	Flexor carpi radialis	15	Flexor retinaculum
12	Pronator teres		

Figure 6-6   Transverse section of the canine left forelimb just distal to the shoulder joint

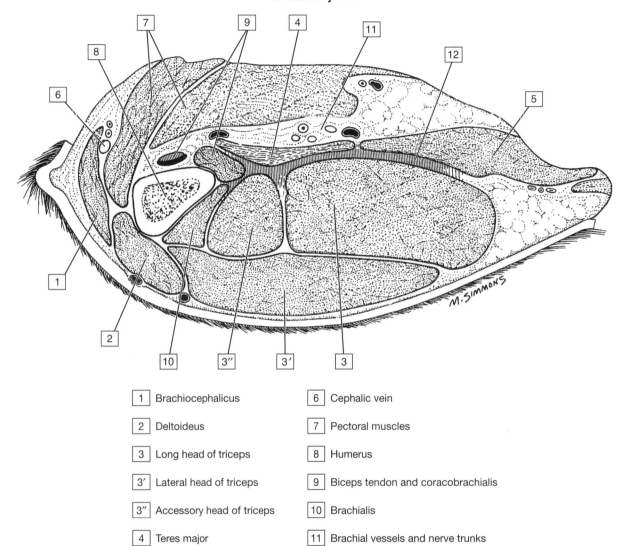

1	Brachiocephalicus	6	Cephalic vein
2	Deltoideus	7	Pectoral muscles
3	Long head of triceps	8	Humerus
3'	Lateral head of triceps	9	Biceps tendon and coracobrachialis
3"	Accessory head of triceps	10	Brachialis
4	Teres major	11	Brachial vessels and nerve trunks
5	Latissimus dorsi	12	Heavy intermuscular fascia

Figure 6-7   Superficial veins on the canine left forearm

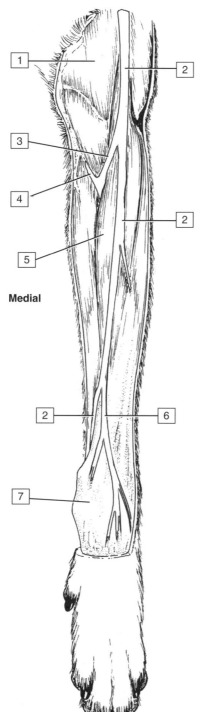

Medial

1	Brachiocephalicus
2	Cephalic v.
3	Median cubital v.
4	Brachial v.
5	Extensor carpi radialis
6	Accessory cephalic v.
7	Carpus

Figure 6-8   Transverse section of the canine left forelimb just proximal to
the carpus

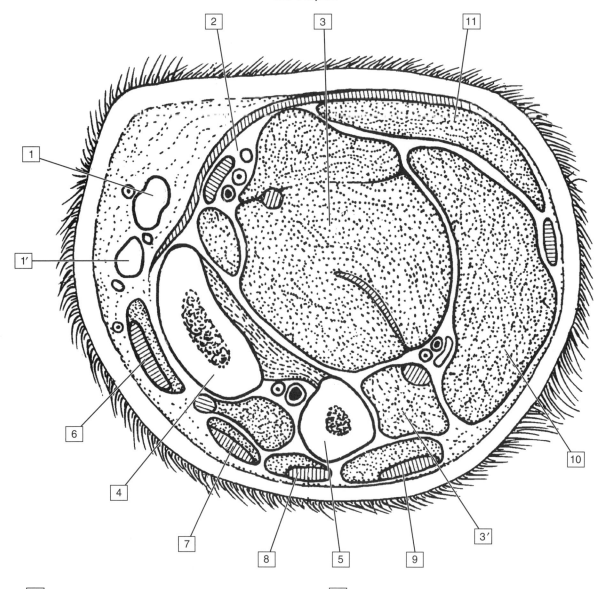

1	Cephalic vein and branches of superficial radial nerve	6	Extensor carpi radialis
1′	Accessory cephalic vein	7	Common digital extensor
2	Median vessels and nerve, and flexor carpi radialis	8	Lateral digital extensor
3	Humeral head of deep digital flexor	9	Ulnaris lateralis
3′	Ulnar head of deep digital flexor	10	Flexor carpi ulnaris: its small ulnar head lies on its caudal aspect, and the ulnar vessels and nerve on its cranial aspect
4	Radius		
5	Ulna	11	Superficial digital flexor

Figure 6-9   Topography of the major arteries of the canine right forelimb,
medial view

The caudomedial muscles of the forearm have been removed.

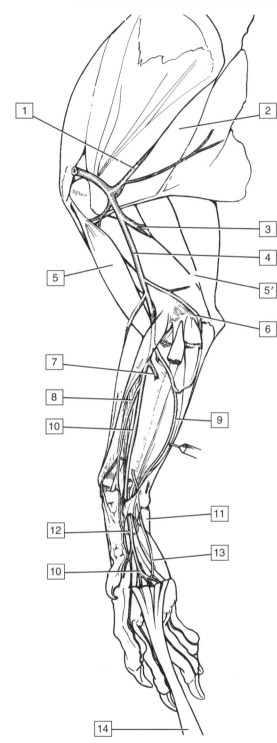

1	Subscapular a.
2	Teres major
3	Deep brachial a.
4	Brachial a.
5	Biceps
5'	Triceps
6	Collateral ulnar a.
7	Deep antebrachial a.
8	Radial a.
9	Ulnar a.
10	Median a.
11	Accessory carpal bone
12	Deep palmar arch
13	Superficial palmar arch
14	Superficial digital flexor, reflected

Figure 6-10 The blood supply of a canine long bone

The supply of the cortex is shown (enlarged) in the center.

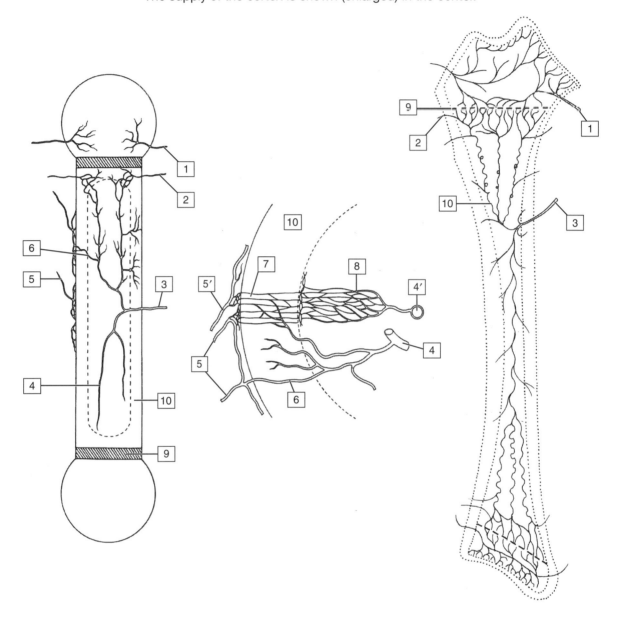

1 Epiphysial aa.	6 Anastomosis between periosteal and bone marrow aa.
2 Metaphysial aa.	7 Capillaries of the cortex
3 Nutrient a.	8 Sinusoids in the bone marrow
4 Artery of the bone marrow	9 Growth cartilage
4' Vein of the bone marrow	10 Cortex
5 Periosteal aa.	
5' Periosteal v.	

Saunders Veterinary Anatomy Coloring Book
Copyright © 2011 by Saunders, an imprint of Elsevier Inc.

Figure 6-11   Cranial view of the canine left stifle joint

The joint is resected to show intra- and extracapsular ligaments.

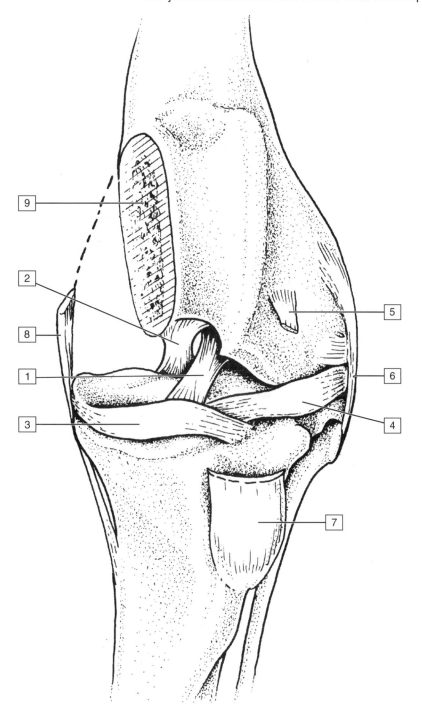

1 | Cranial cruciate ligament

2 | Caudal cruciate ligament

3 | Medial meniscus

4 | Lateral meniscus

5 | Tendon of origin of long digital extensor

6 | Lateral collateral ligament

7 | Patellar ligament

8 | Medial collateral ligament

9 | Medial condyle, partly removed

Figure 6-12   Sections of a synovial bursa (*A*) and a tendon sheath (*B*)

The bursa permits frictionless movement of a tendon over bone, the sheath movement of a tendon over bone and under a retinaculum, respectively. The arrows show that a tendon sheath may be regarded as a large bursa that has wrapped around a tendon.

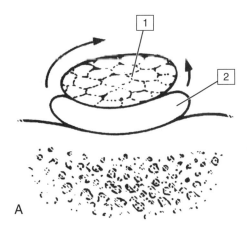

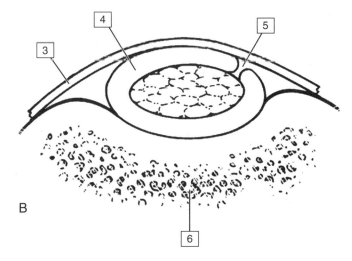

1	Tendon	5	Mesotendon, through which blood vessels reach the tendon
2	Bursa	6	Bone
3	Retinaculum		
4	Tendon sheath		

Figure 6-13   Canine left forelimb skeleton, lateral view of muscle attachments

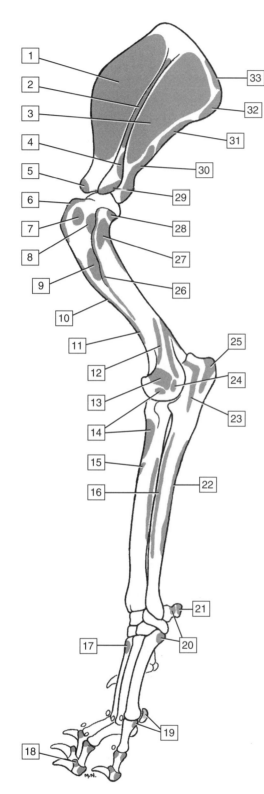

1 Supraspinatus

2 Trapezius and deltoideus

3 Infraspinatus

4 Omotransversarius

5 Biceps brachii

6 Supraspinatus

7 Infraspinatus

8 Teres minor

9 Deltoideus

10 Superficial pectorals

11 Cleidobrachialis

12 Extensor carpi radialis

13 Extensors of carpus and digits

14 Supinator

15 Pronator teres

16 Abductor digiti I longus

17 Extensor carpi radialis

18 Lateral and common digital extensors

19 Interossei

20 Ulnaris lateralis

21 Flexor carpi ulnaris

22 Deep digital flexor

23 Anconeus

24 Ulnaris lateralis

25 Triceps

26 Anconeus

27 Brachialis

28 Triceps, accessory head

29 Deltoideus

30 Triceps, long head and teres minor

31 Subscapularis

32 Teres major

33 Rhomboideus

Figure 6-14   Major extensors and flexors of the canine left forelimb

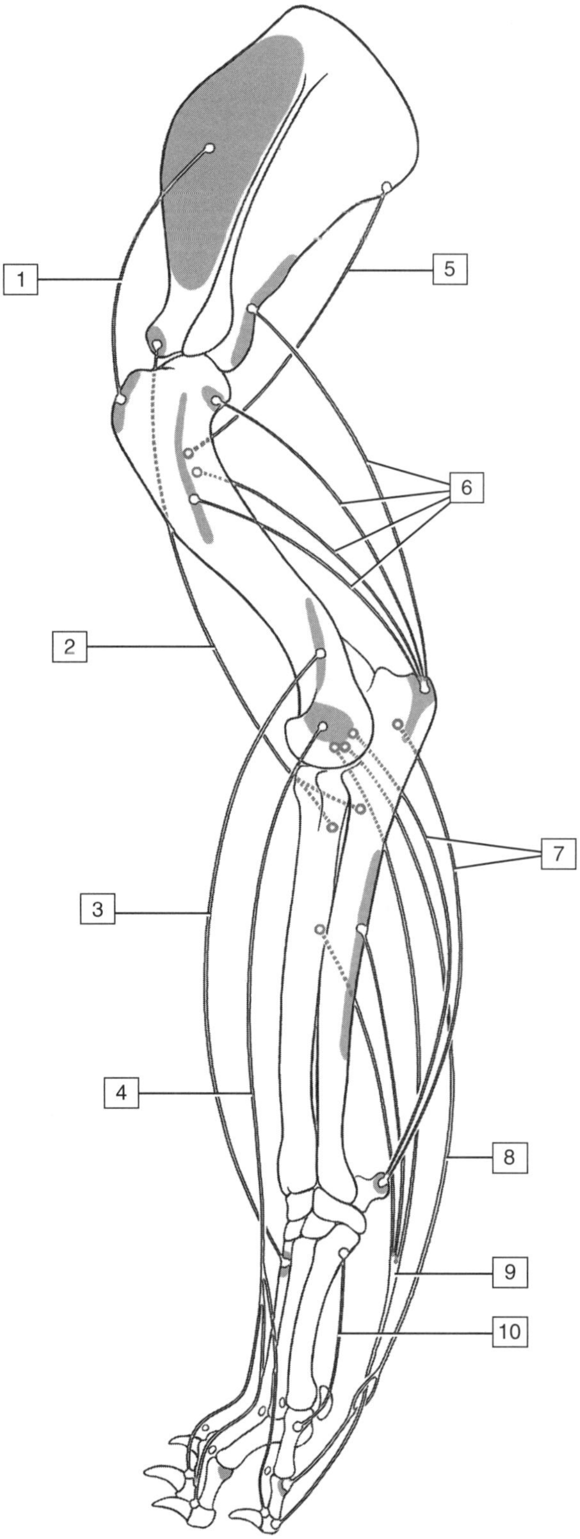

1   Supraspinatus

2   Biceps

3   Extensor carpi radialis

4   Common digital extensor

5   Teres major

6   Triceps, four heads

7   Flexor carpi ulnaris, two heads

8   Superficial digital flexor

9   Deep digital flexor, three heads

10 Interosseus

Saunders Veterinary Anatomy Coloring Book
Copyright © 2011 by Saunders, an imprint of Elsevier Inc.

Figure 6-15 *A,* Distribution of canine musculocutaneous and median nerves, right forelimb, medial view. *B,* Distribution of canine radial nerve, right forelimb, lateral view.

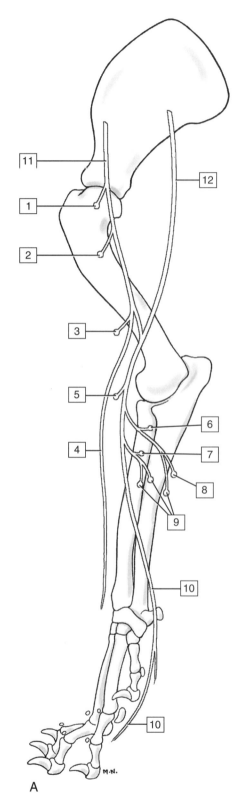

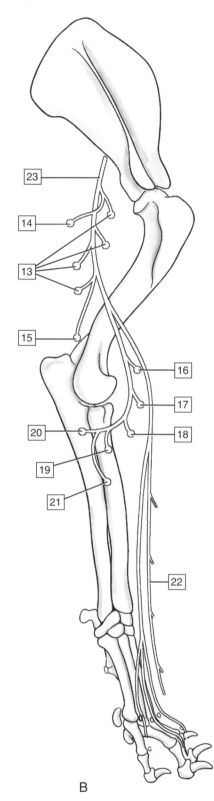

Musculocutaneous nerve

1 Coracobrachialis

2 Biceps brachii

3 Brachialis

4 Skin of medial antebrachium

Median nerve

5 Pronator teres

6 Flexor carpi radialis

7 Pronator quadratus

8 Superficial digital flexor

9 Deep digital flexor, humeral, ulnar, and radial heads

10 Skin of caudal antebrachium and palmar paw

11 Musculocutaneous nerve

12 Median nerve

Radial nerve

13 Triceps brachii

14 Tensor fasciae antebrachii

15 Anconeus

16 Extensor carpi radialis

17 Supinator

18 Common digital extensor

19 Lateral digital extensor

20 Ulnaris lateralis

21 Abductor digiti I longus

22 Skin of cranial and lateral antebrachium and dorsal paw

23 Radial nerve

Figure 6-16   Distribution of canine ulnar nerve, right forelimb, medial view

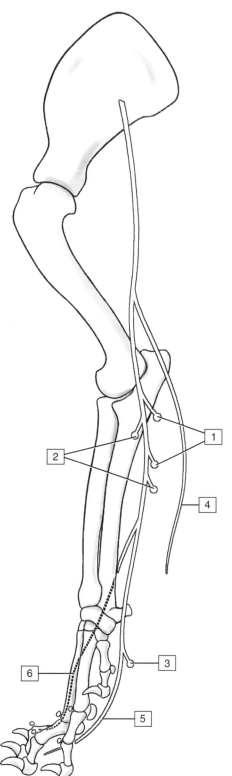

1	Flexor carpi ulnaris, ulnar and humeral heads
2	Deep digital flexor, ulnar and humeral heads
3	Interossei
4	Skin of caudal antebrachium
5	Skin of palmar paw
6	Skin of fifth metacarpal, lateral surface of digit

Saunders Veterinary Anatomy Coloring Book
Copyright © 2011 by Saunders, an imprint of Elsevier Inc.

Figure 6-17   Veins of canine right forelimb, schematic medial view

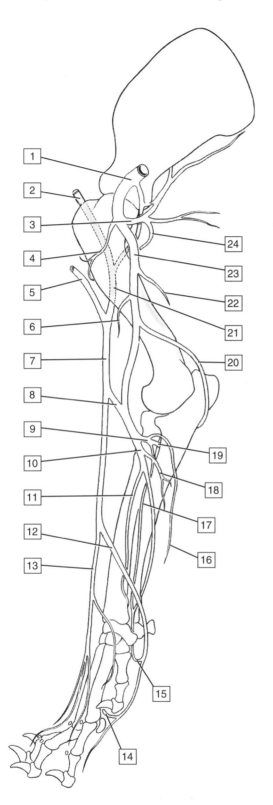

1	Axillary
2	Omobrachial to external jugular
3	Subscapular
4	Cranial circumflex humeral
5	Cephalic to external jugular
6	Bicipital
7	Cephalic
8	Median cubital
9	Common interosseous
10	Median
11	Radial
12	Cephalic
13	Accessory cephalic
14	Distal palmar venous arch
15	Proximal palmar venous arch
16	Ulnar
17	Caudal interosseous
18	Deep antebrachial
19	Cranial interosseous
20	Collateral ulnar
21	Axillobrachial
22	Deep brachial
23	Brachial
24	Caudal circumflex humeral

Figure 6-18   Equine superficial muscles and veins

The cutaneous muscles except for the cutaneous colli have been removed.

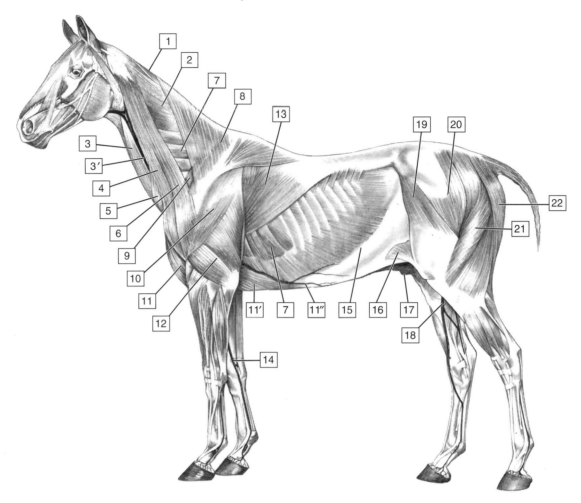

1 Rhomboideus	9 Subclavius	16 Stump of cutaneus trunci forming flank fold
2 Splenius	10 Deltoideus	17 Sheath
3 Sternocephalicus	11 Pectoralis descendens	18 Medial saphenous vein
3′ Jugular vein	11′ Pectoralis ascendens	19 Tensor fasciae latae
4 Brachiocephalicus	11″ Superficial thoracic vein	20 Gluteus superficialis
5 Cutaneous colli	12 Triceps	21 Biceps femoris
6 Omotransversarius	13 Latissimus dorsi	22 Semitendinosus
7 Serratus ventralis	14 Cephalic vein	
8 Trapezius	15 External abdominal oblique	

Saunders Veterinary Anatomy Coloring Book
Copyright © 2011 by Saunders, an imprint of Elsevier Inc.

Figure 6-19   Muscles on the ventral surface of the equine thorax

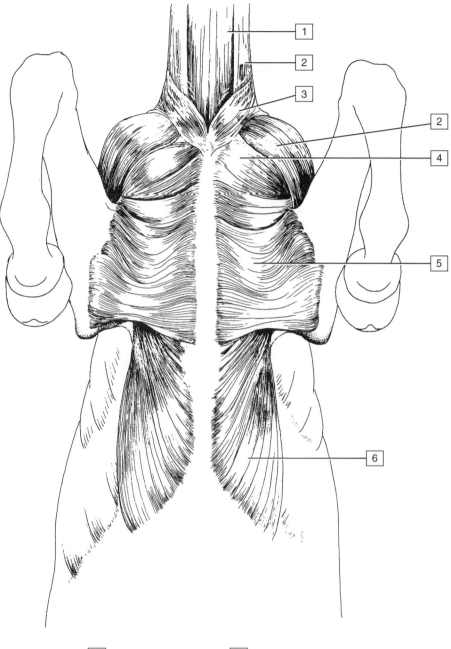

1	Sternocephalicus	4	Pectoralis descendens
2	Brachiocephalicus	5	Pectoralis transversus
3	Cutaneus colli	6	Pectoralis profundus

Figure 6-20   Deep muscles attaching the equine forelimb to the trunk

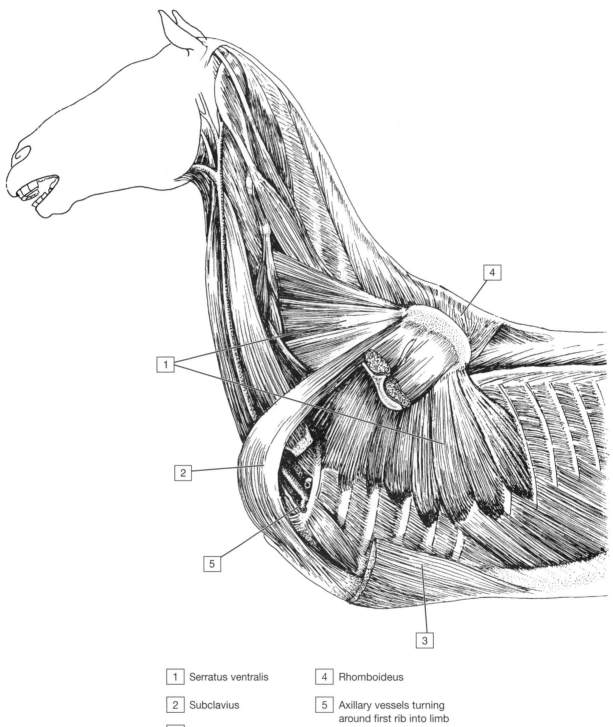

1	Serratus ventralis	4	Rhomboideus
2	Subclavius	5	Axillary vessels turning around first rib into limb
3	Pectoralis profundus		

Saunders Veterinary Anatomy Coloring Book
Copyright © 2011 by Saunders, an imprint of Elsevier Inc.

Figure 6-21   Muscles associated with the equine shoulder and elbow joints, lateral view

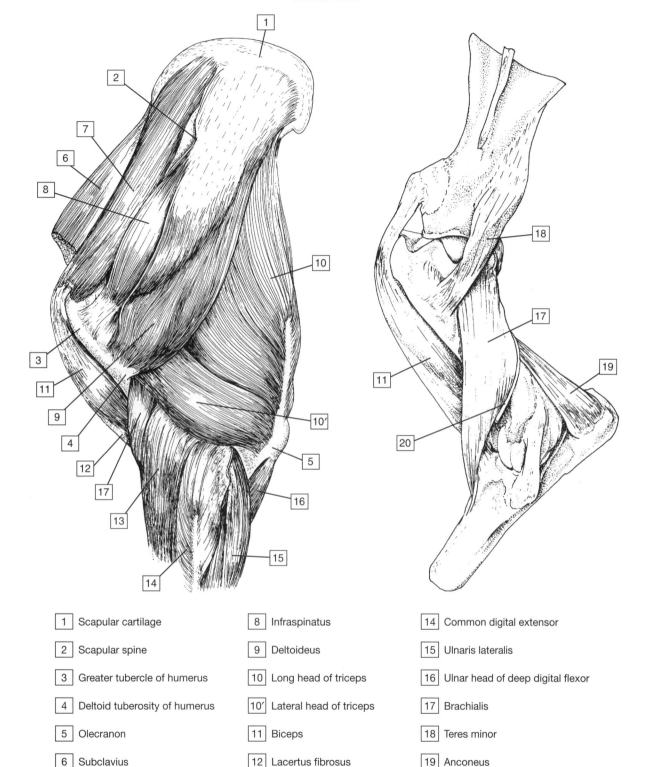

1 Scapular cartilage	8 Infraspinatus	14 Common digital extensor
2 Scapular spine	9 Deltoideus	15 Ulnaris lateralis
3 Greater tubercle of humerus	10 Long head of triceps	16 Ulnar head of deep digital flexor
4 Deltoid tuberosity of humerus	10' Lateral head of triceps	17 Brachialis
5 Olecranon	11 Biceps	18 Teres minor
6 Subclavius	12 Lacertus fibrosus	19 Anconeus
7 Supraspinatus	13 Extensor carpi radialis	20 Radial nerve

Figure 6-22   Nerves and arteries on the medial surface of the equine right
shoulder and arm

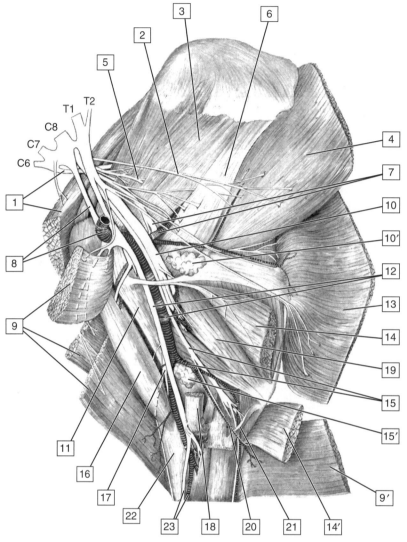

1	Suprascapular n. and subclavius	
2	Thoracodorsal n.	
3	Subscapularis	
4	Latissimus dorsi	
5	Subscapular n.	
6	Teres major	
7	Axillary n. and subscapular a.	
8	Musculocutaneous n. and axillary a.	
9	Pectoralis profundus	
9′	Pectoralis descendens	

9″	Pectoralis transversus
10	Radial n.
10′	Axillary lymph nodes
11	Coracobrachialis
12	Median n. and brachial a.
13	Cutaneus trunci
14	Stump of tensor fasciae antebrachii
14′	Stump of tensor fasciae antebrachii
15	Ulnar n. and collateral ulnar a.

15′	Cubital lymph nodes
16	Biceps
17	Musculocutaneous and medial cutaneous antebrachial nn.
18	Flexor carpi radialis
19	Triceps
20	Caudal cutaneous antebrachial n.
21	Flexor carpi ulnaris
22	Lacertus fibrosus
23	Median n. and a.

Figure 6-23   Distal muscles of the equine left forelimb, medial view

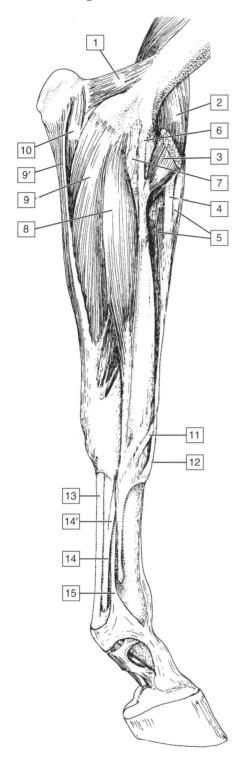

1	Anconeus
2	Brachialis
3	Biceps
4	Lacertus fibrosus
5	Extensor carpi radialis
6	Long part of medial collateral ligament (pronator teres)
7	Short part of medial collateral ligament
8	Flexor carpi radialis
9	Humeral and ulnar heads of flexor carpi ulnaris
9′	Humeral and ulnar heads of flexor carpi ulnaris
10	Ulnar head of deep digital flexor
11	Tendon of extensor carpi obliquus
12	Tendon of extensor carpi radialis
13	Tendon of superficial digital flexor
14	Tendon of deep digital flexor
14′	Accessory (check) ligament
15	Interosseus

Figure 6-24   Skeleton of the distal part of the equine left forelimb,
dorsal view

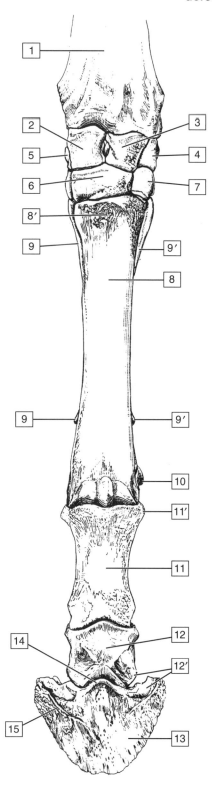

1	Radius
2	Radial carpal
3	Intermediate carpal
4	Ulnar carpal
5	Second carpal
6	Third carpal
7	Fourth carpal
8	Large metacarpal bone
8′	Metacarpal tuberosity
9	Medial splint bone
9′	Lateral splint bone
10	Proximal sesamoid bones
11	Proximal phalanx
11′	Proximal tubercle
12	Middle phalanx
12′	Attachments of collateral ligament of coffin joint
13	Distal phalanx
14	Extensor process
15	Parietal groove

Figure 6-25   Axial section of equine digit

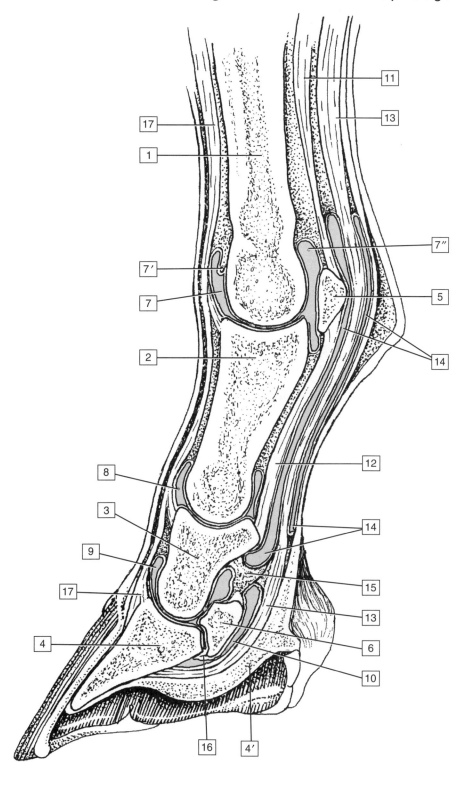

1	Large metacarpal bone
2	Proximal phalanx
3	Middle phalanx
4	Distal phalanx
4'	Digital cushion
5	Proximal sesamoid bone
6	Distal sesamoid (navicular) bone
7	Dorsal pouch of fetlock joint
7'	Capsular fold
7"	Palmar pouch of fetlock joint
8	Dorsal pouch of pastern and coffin joints
9	Dorsal pouch of pastern and coffin joints
10	Navicular bursa
11	Interosseus
12	Straight sesamoidean ligament
13	Deep flexor tendon
14	Digital sheath
15	Connective tissue bridge
16	Distal navicular ligament
17	Common digital extensor tendon

Figure 6-26   The major arteries of the equine right forelimb, palmar view

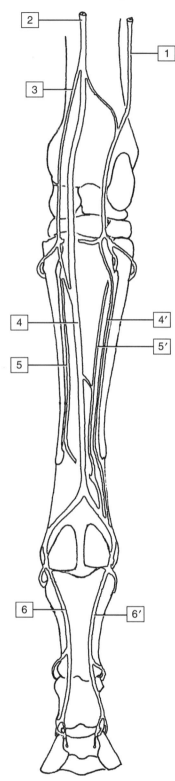

1	Collateral ulnar a.
2	Median a.
3	Radial a.
4	Medial a.
4'	Lateral palmar a.
5	Medial palmar metacarpal a.
5'	Lateral palmar metacarpal a.
6	Medial digital a.
6'	Lateral digital a.

Figure 6-27   Transverse section of the equine left elbow

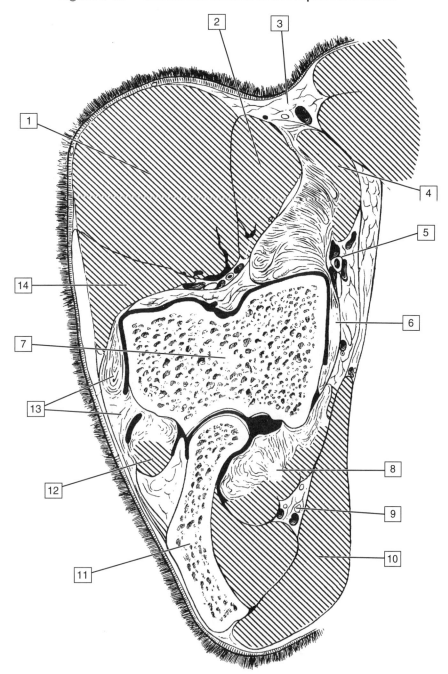

1 Extensor carpi radialis	6 Medial collateral ligament	11 Olecranon
2 Brachialis	7 Humerus	12 Ulnaris lateralis
3 Medial cutaneous antebrachial nerve and cephalic vein lying on lacertus fibrosus	8 Flexors arising from medial epicondyle of humerus	13 Lateral collateral ligament
4 Biceps	9 Ulnar nerve and collateral ulnar vessels	14 Common digital extensor
5 Brachial vessels and median nerve	10 Tensor fasciae antebrachii	

Figure 6-28   Transverse section of the middle of the bovine left forearm

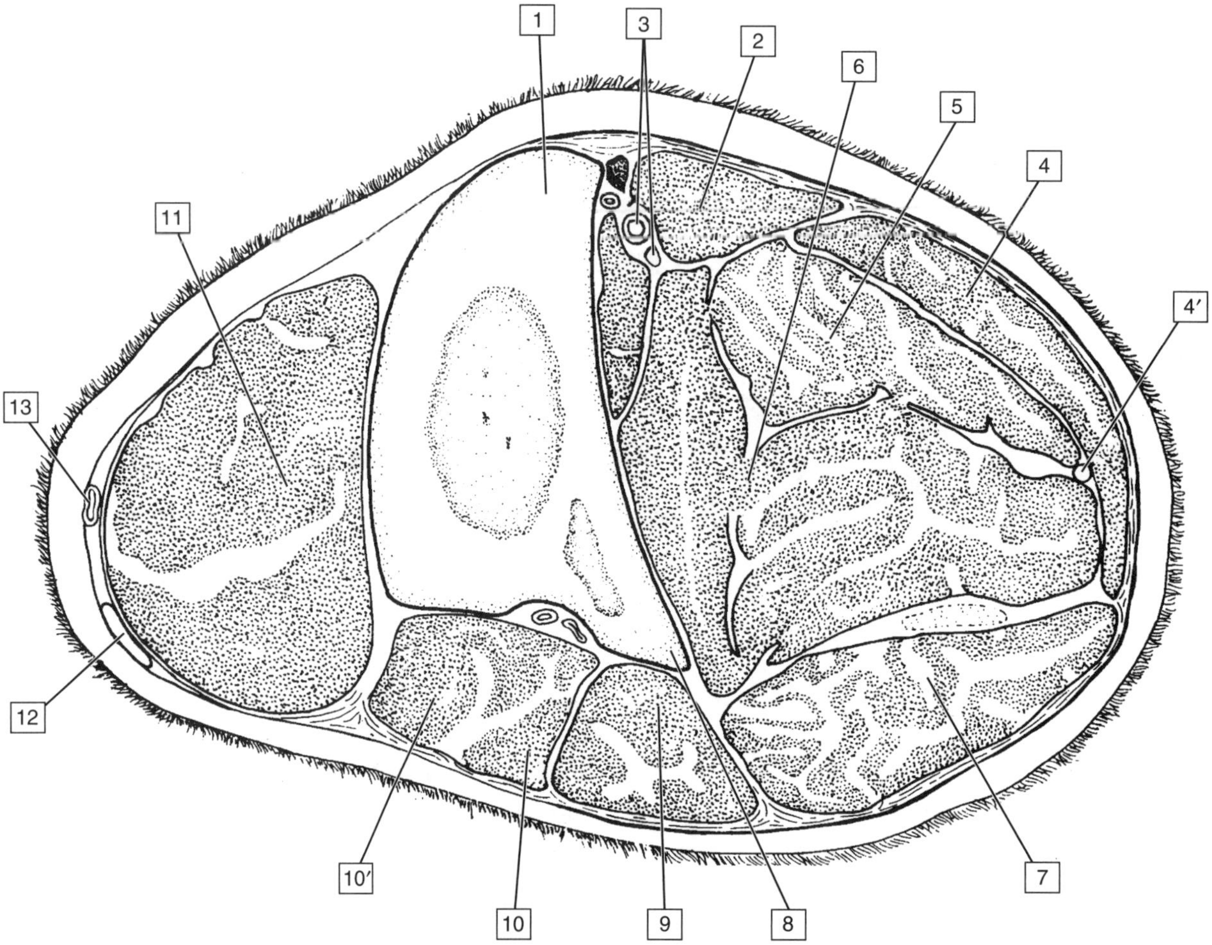

1	Radius	8	Ulna
2	Flexor carpi radialis	9	Lateral digital extensor
3	Median vessels and nerve	10	Common digital extensor
4	Flexor carpi ulnaris	10'	Common digital extensor
4'	Ulnar nerve	11	Extensor carpi radialis
5	Superficial digital flexor	12	Superficial branch of radial nerve
6	Deep digital flexor	13	Cephalic vein
7	Ulnaris lateralis		

THE FORELIMB 6
Figure 6-29   Sagittal section of the bovine foot, splitting the lateral digit

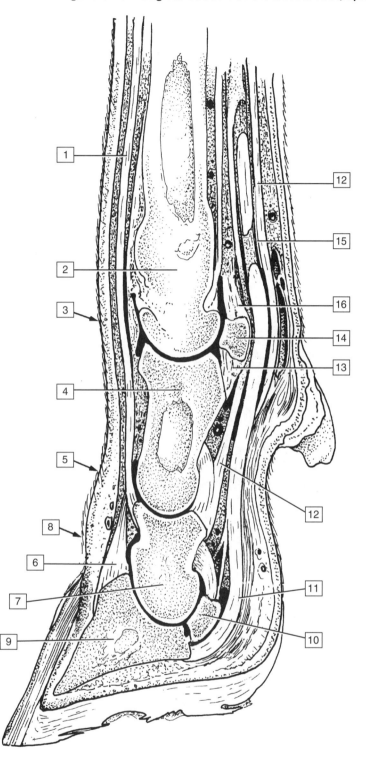

1 Lateral digital extensor
2 Metacarpal bone
3 Fetlock joint
4 Proximal phalanx
5 Pastern joint
6 Common digital extensor
7 Middle phalanx
8 Coffin joint
9 Distal phalanx
10 Navicular bone
11 Deep digital flexor
12 Superficial flexor
13 Distal sesamoidean ligaments
14 Proximal sesamoid bone
15 Digital sheath
16 Interosseus

Figure 6-30   Sagittal section of the medial digit of the bovine forefoot

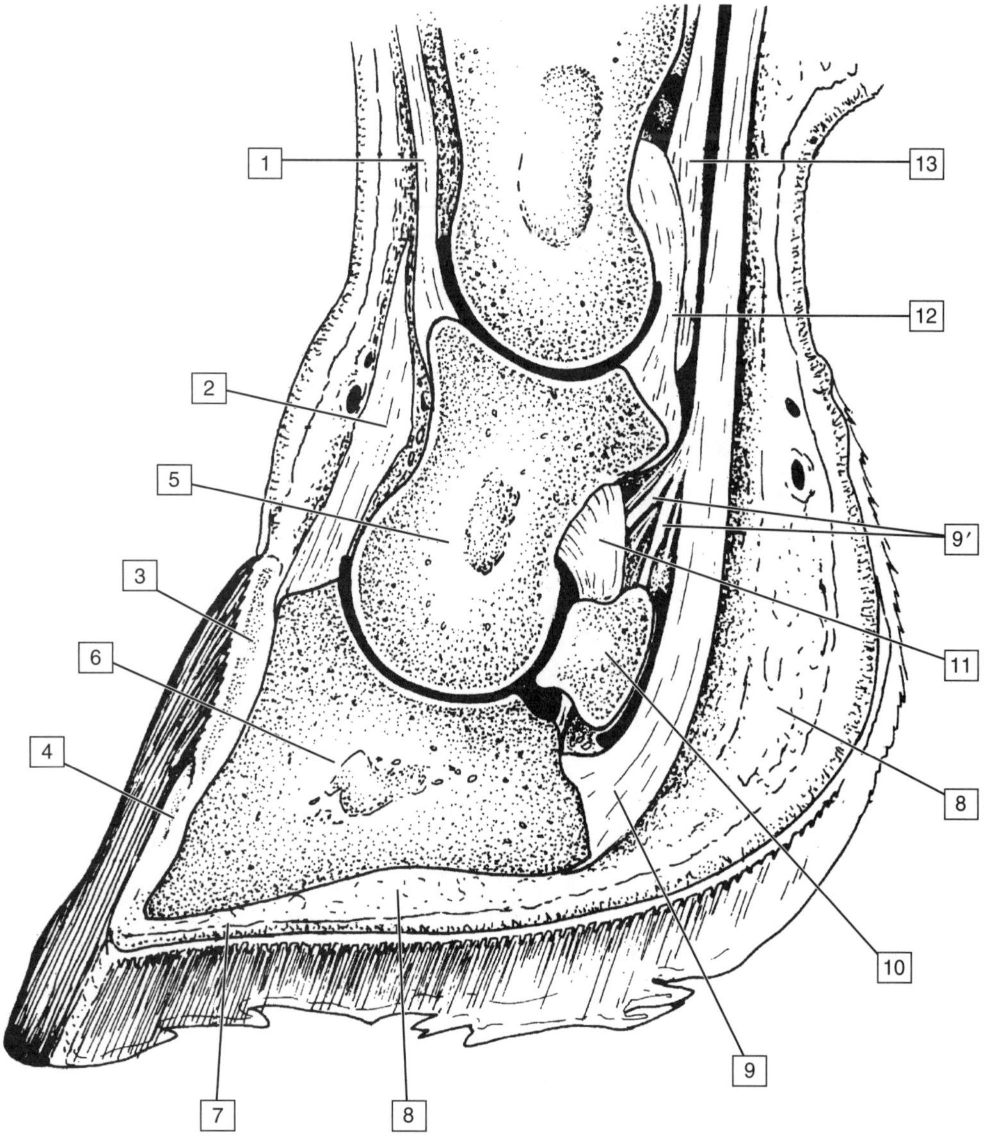

1 Proper (medial) digital extensor	**9** Deep digital flexor
2 Common digital extensor	**9′** Fibers of deep digital flexor to the middle phalanx and navicular bone
3 Coronary dermis	**10** Navicular bone
4 Laminar dermis	**11** Collateral navicular ligament
5 Middle phalanx	**12** Palmar ligaments of pastern joint
6 Distal phalanx	**13** Superficial digital flexor
7 Sole dermis covered by sole	
8 Digital cushion	

Figure 6-31   Dermis over which the horny bovine hoof is produced, abaxial
and ground surface

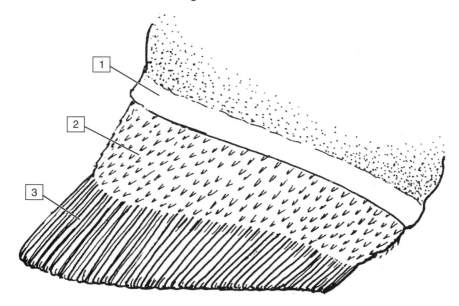

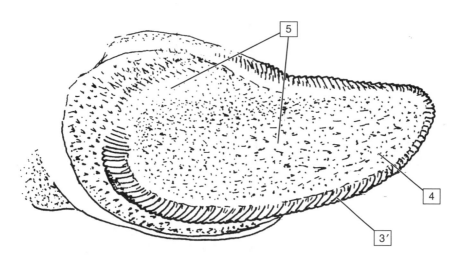

1	Perioplic dermis	3'	Terminal papillae at the distal ends of the laminae
2	Coronary dermis	4	Sole dermis
3	Laminar dermis	5	Dermis of the bulb

Figure 6-32   The principal veins of the bovine forelimb

A, Left foot, lateral view. *B*, Right foot, dorsal view.

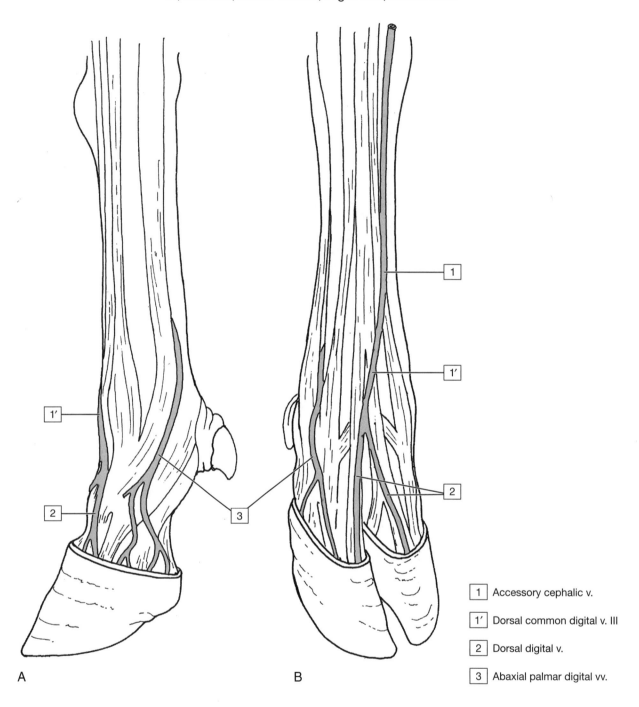

A   B

1	Accessory cephalic v.
1′	Dorsal common digital v. III
2	Dorsal digital v.
3	Abaxial palmar digital vv.

Figure 6-33   The principal nerves of the bovine right forefoot in lateral and dorsal views

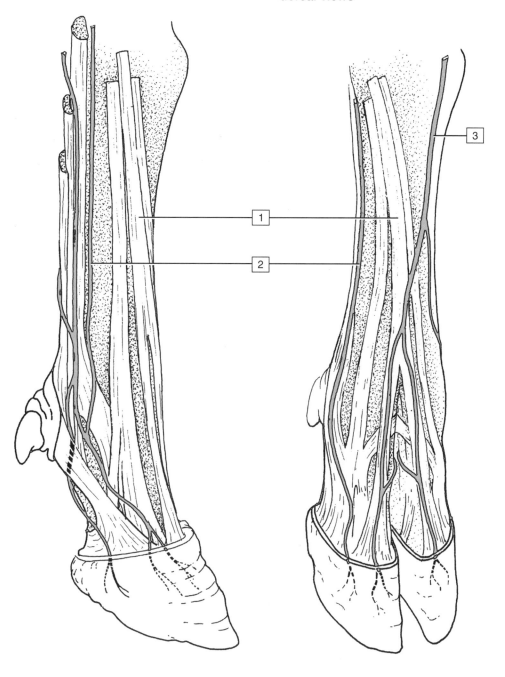

| 1 | Digital extensor tendons |

| 2 | Dorsal branch of ulnar n. |

| 3 | Superficial branch of radial n. |

Figure 6-34   Left porcine forefoot, caudomedial view

Inset shows the carpal glands on the undersurface of the skin, enlarged.

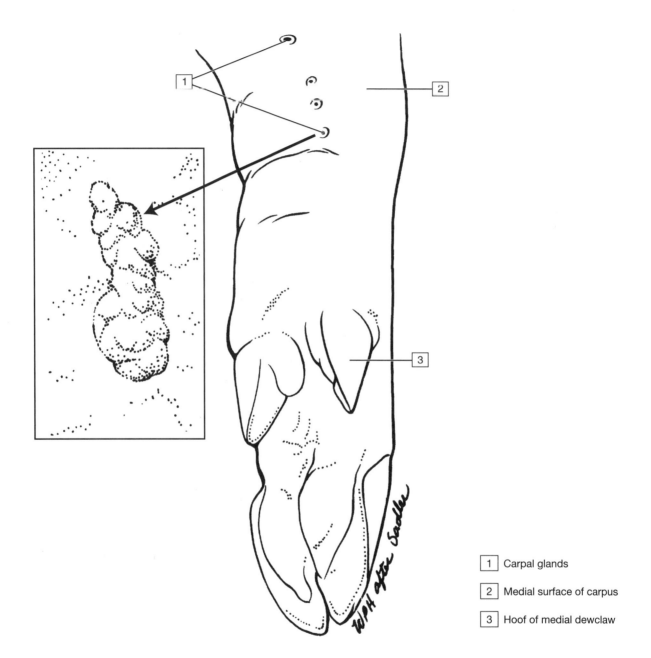

1	Carpal glands
2	Medial surface of carpus
3	Hoof of medial dewclaw

Figure 6-35   Skeleton of avian left wing, partially extended laterally

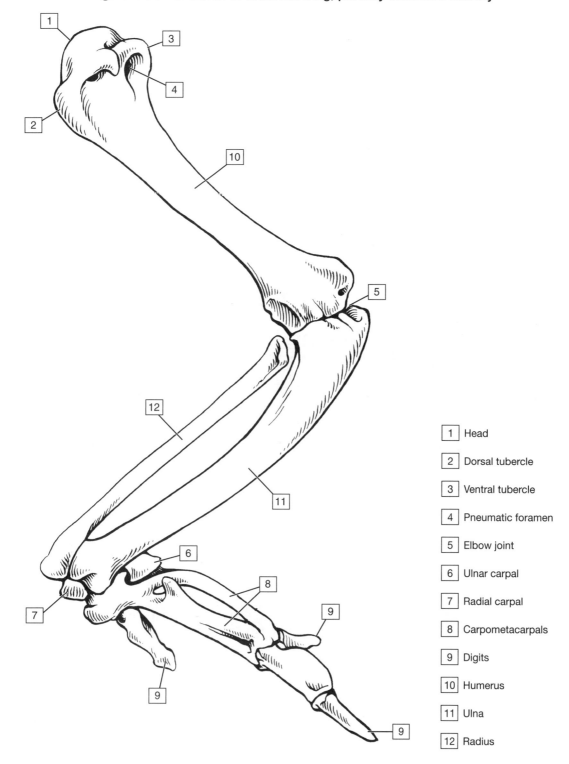

1	Head
2	Dorsal tubercle
3	Ventral tubercle
4	Pneumatic foramen
5	Elbow joint
6	Ulnar carpal
7	Radial carpal
8	Carpometacarpals
9	Digits
10	Humerus
11	Ulna
12	Radius

Figure 6-36   Superficial dissection of laterally extended avian left wing,
ventral surface

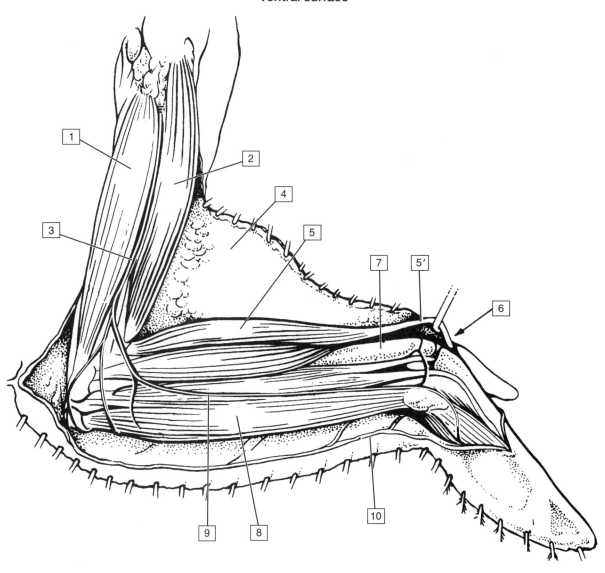

1	Triceps	6	Carpal joint
2	Biceps	7	Subcutaneous part of radius
3	Brachial vein	8	Flexor carpi ulnaris
4	Skin fold (propatagium)	9	Cutaneous ulnar (wing) vein
5	Extensor carpi radialis	10	Reflected skin
5'	Tendon of extensor carpi radialis		

FIGURE 6-37 Bones of the carpal skeleton

Carnivores (*Car*), horse (*eq*), cattle (*bo*), and pig (*su*), schematic.
Roman numerals identify the metacarpal bones.

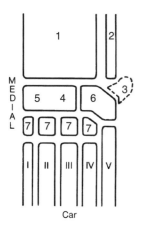 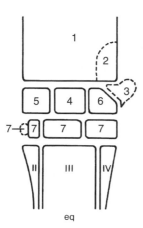 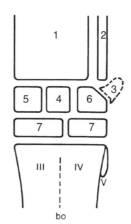 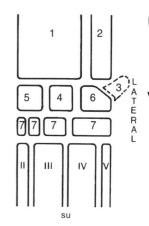

1 Radius	5 Radial carpal bone	
2 Ulna	6 Ulnar carpal bone	
3 Accessory carpal bone	7 Distal carpal bones	
4 Intermediate carpal bone		

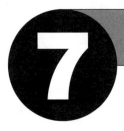

Figure 7-1   Skeleton of canine right pes, dorsal view

Roman numerals identify the metatarsal bones.

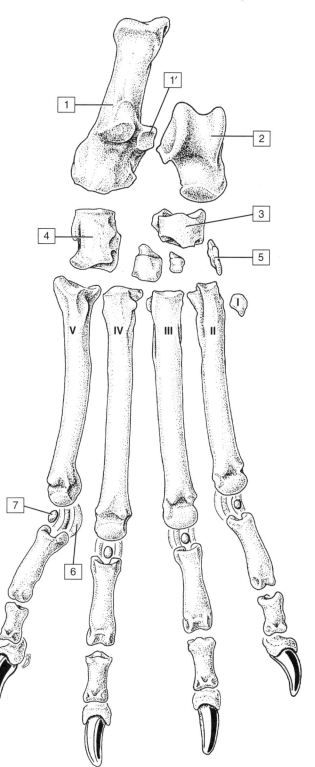

1	Calcaneus
1'	Sustentaculum tali
2	Talus
3	Central tarsal
4	Fourth tarsal
5	First, second, and third tarsal bones in distal row
6	Proximal sesamoid bones
7	Dorsal sesamoid bones

Figure 7-2 Canine left stifle joint, cranial views (*A-C*)

The extent of the joint capsule is shown in *B*. The patella has been removed in *C*.

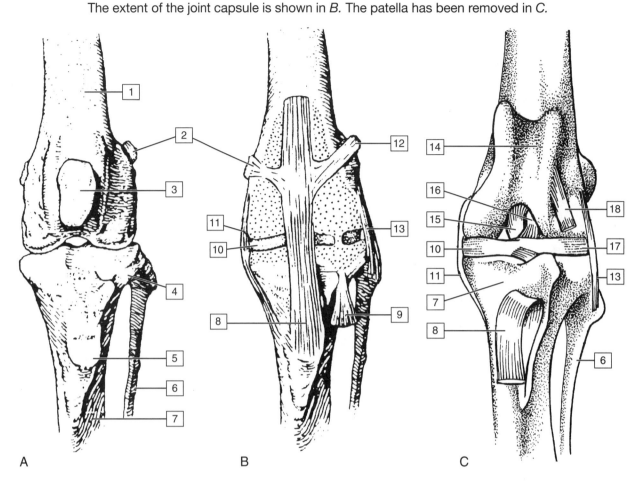

A   B   C

1	Femur	10	Medial meniscus
2	Sesamoids in gastrocnemius	11	Medial collateral ligament
3	Patella	12	Lateral femoropatellar ligament
4	Extensor groove	13	Lateral collateral ligament
5	Tibial tuberosity	14	Trochlea
6	Fibula	15	Caudal cruciate ligament
7	Tibia	16	Cranial cruciate ligament
8	Patellar ligament	17	Lateral meniscus
9	Tendon of long digital extensor passing through extensor groove	18	Stump of 9

Saunders Veterinary Anatomy Coloring Book

Figure 7-3 Muscles of the canine hindquarter and thigh, lateral (*A*) and medial (*B*) views

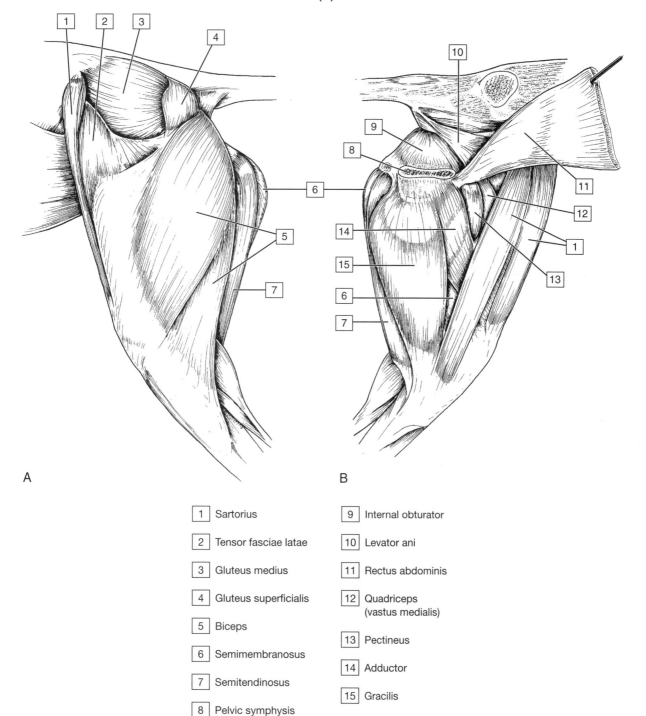

A

B

1 Sartorius	9 Internal obturator
2 Tensor fasciae latae	10 Levator ani
3 Gluteus medius	11 Rectus abdominis
4 Gluteus superficialis	12 Quadriceps (vastus medialis)
5 Biceps	13 Pectineus
6 Semimembranosus	14 Adductor
7 Semitendinosus	15 Gracilis
8 Pelvic symphysis	

Figure 7-4   Muscles of the canine left leg, lateral and medial views

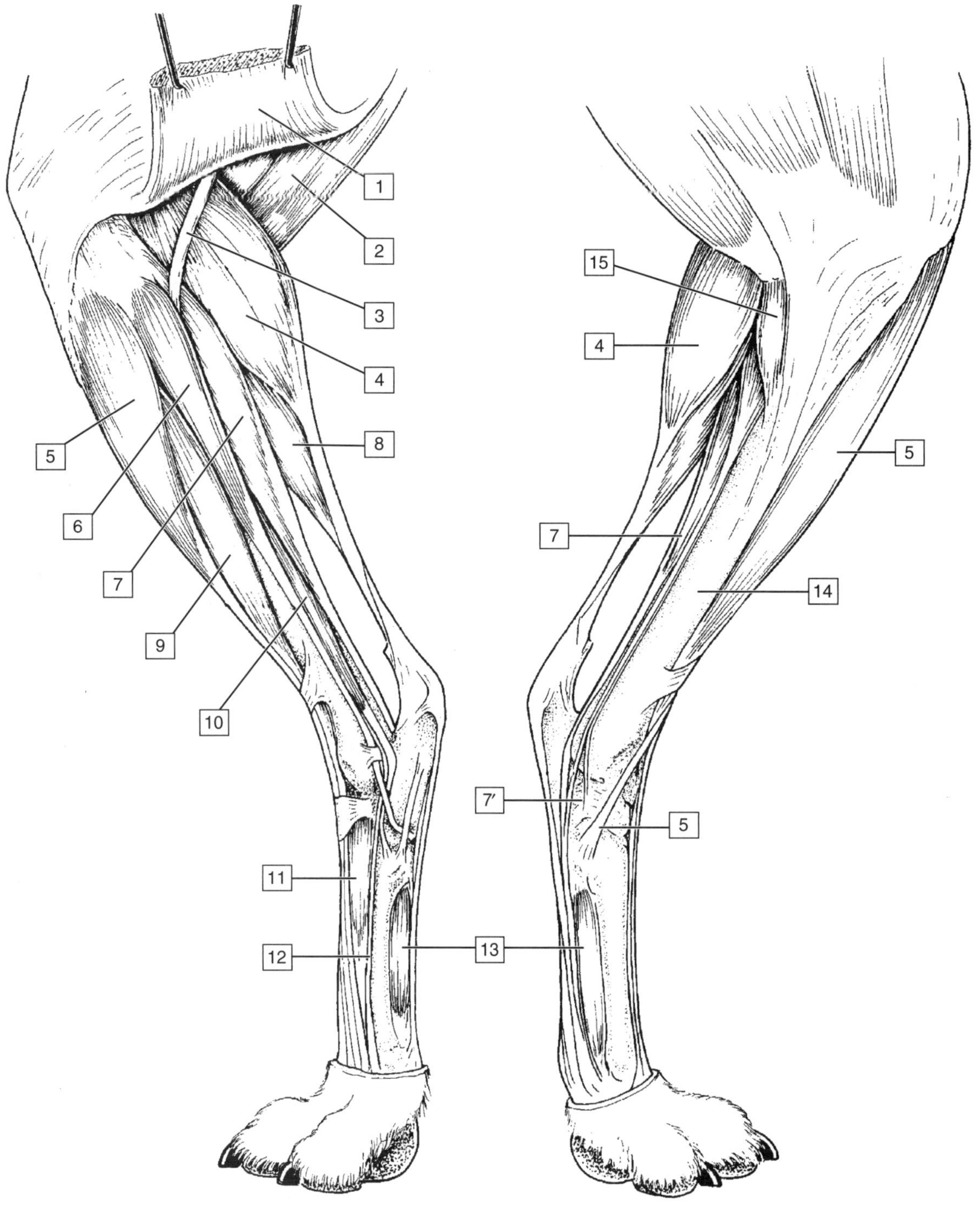

1	Biceps	6	Peroneus longus
2	Semitendinosus	7	Lateral deep digital flexor
3	Peroneal nerve	7′	Tendon of the smaller medial deep digital flexor
4	Gastrocnemius	8	Superficial digital flexor
5	Tibialis cranialis		

9	Long digital extensor	13	Interossei
10	Peroneus brevis	14	Tibia
11	Extensor brevis	15	Popliteus
12	Tendon of lateral digital extensor		

Figure 7-5   Transverse section of the canine left thigh

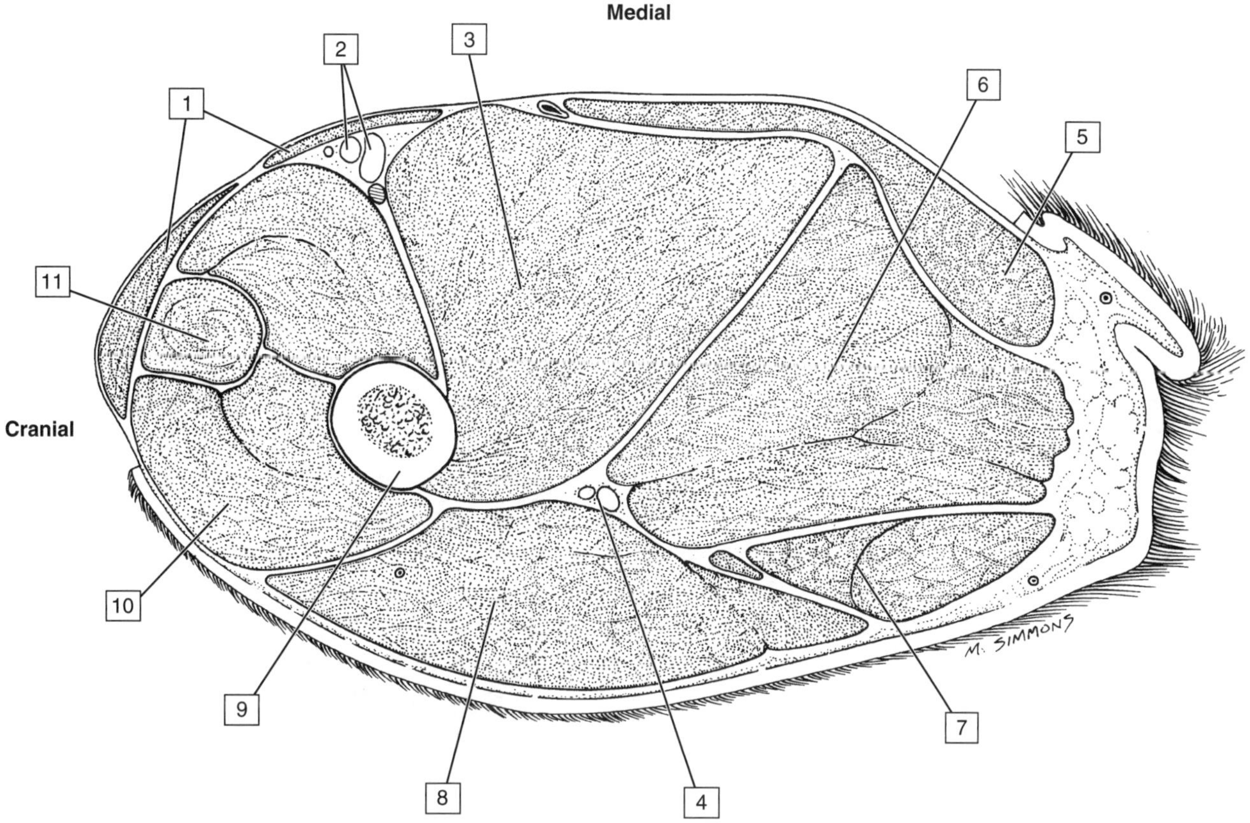

Medial

Cranial

M. SIMMONS

1	Sartorius	7	Semitendinosus
2	Femoral vessels	8	Biceps
3	Adductor	9	Femur
4	Sciatic nerve	10	Vastus lateralis (of quadriceps)
5	Gracilis	11	Rectus femoris
6	Semimembranosus		

Figure 7-6   Canine left hindlimb

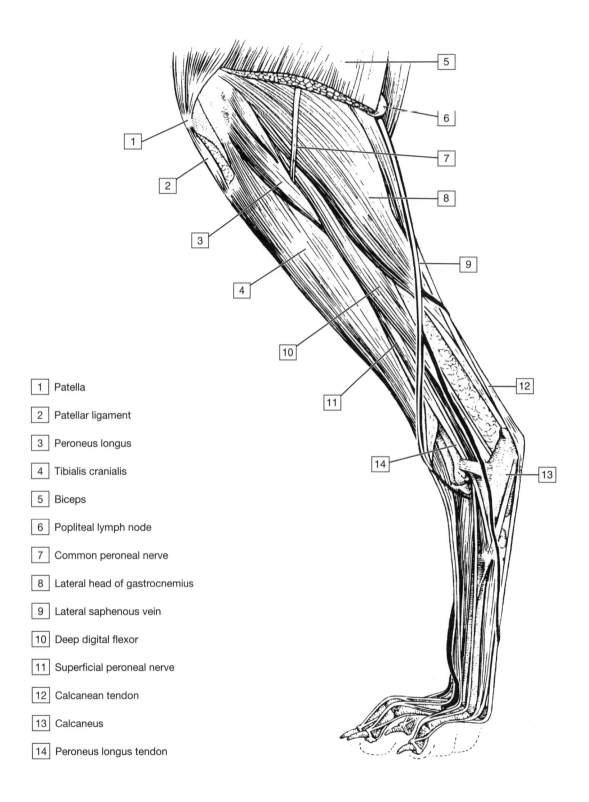

1 Patella

2 Patellar ligament

3 Peroneus longus

4 Tibialis cranialis

5 Biceps

6 Popliteal lymph node

7 Common peroneal nerve

8 Lateral head of gastrocnemius

9 Lateral saphenous vein

10 Deep digital flexor

11 Superficial peroneal nerve

12 Calcanean tendon

13 Calcaneus

14 Peroneus longus tendon

Saunders Veterinary Anatomy Coloring Book

Figure 7-7   Superficial muscles of the canine left pelvic limb, medial view

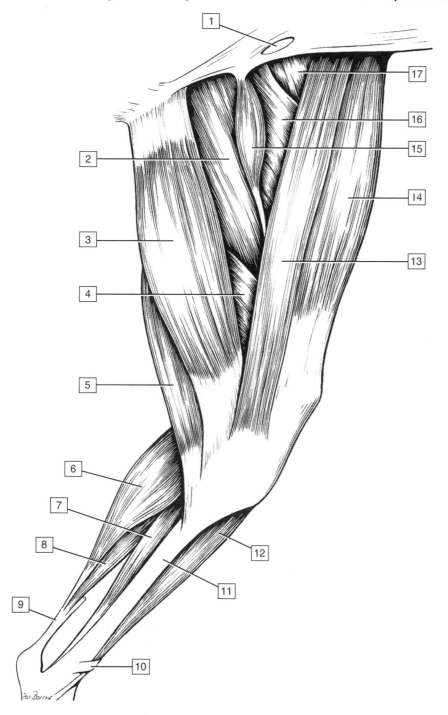

1	Superficial inguinal ring
2	Adductor
3	Gracilis
4	Semimembranosus
5	Semitendinosus
6	Gastrocnemius
7	Lateral digital flexor
8	Superficial digital flexor
9	Common calcaneal tendon
10	Crural extensor retinaculum
11	Tibia
12	Cranial tibial
13	Sartorius, caudal part
14	Sartorius, cranial part
15	Pectineus
16	Vastus medialis
17	Rectus femoris

Figure 7-8   Muscle attachments on the canine pelvis and left pelvic limb, medial view

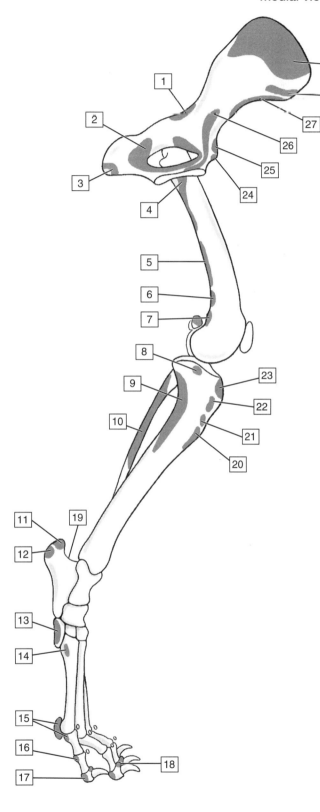

1	Coccygeus
2	Internal obturator
3	Ischiocavernosus
4	Vastus medialis
5	Pectineus
6	Semimembranosus
7	Gastrocnemius
8	Semimembranosus
9	Popliteus
10	Lateral digital flexor
11	Gastrocnemius
12	Superficial digital flexor
13	Cranial tibial
14	Peroneus longus
15	Interosseus
16	Superficial digital flexor
17	Deep digital flexor
18	Long digital flexor
19	Biceps, gracillis and semitendinosus
20	Semitendinosus
21	Gracilis
22	Sartorius
23	Quadriceps
24	Pectineus
25	Psoas minor
26	Levator ani
27	Iliacus
28	Quadratus lumborum
29	Iliocostalis and longissimus lumborum

Saunders Veterinary Anatomy Coloring Book
Copyright © 2011 by Saunders, an imprint of Elsevier Inc.

Figure 7-9   Arteries of the canine right pelvic limb, schematic medial view

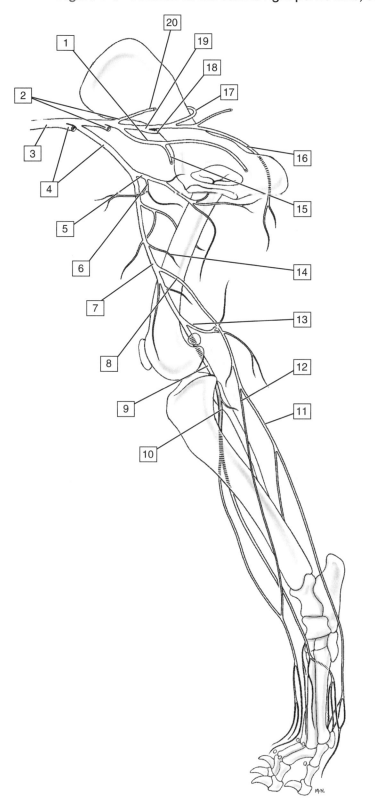

1	Internal pudendal
2	Left and right internal iliac
3	Aorta
4	Left and right external iliac
5	Deep femoral
6	Pudendoepigastric trunk
7	Femoral
8	Saphenous
9	Popliteal
10	Cranial tibial
11	Caudal branch of saphenous
12	Cranial branch of saphenous
13	Distal caudal femoral
14	Proximal caudal femoral
15	Prostatic/vaginal
16	Caudal gluteal
17	Cranial gluteal
18	Iliolumbar
19	Caudal gluteal
20	Median sacral

Figure 7-10   Arteries and nerves of the canine right thigh and crus,
lateral view

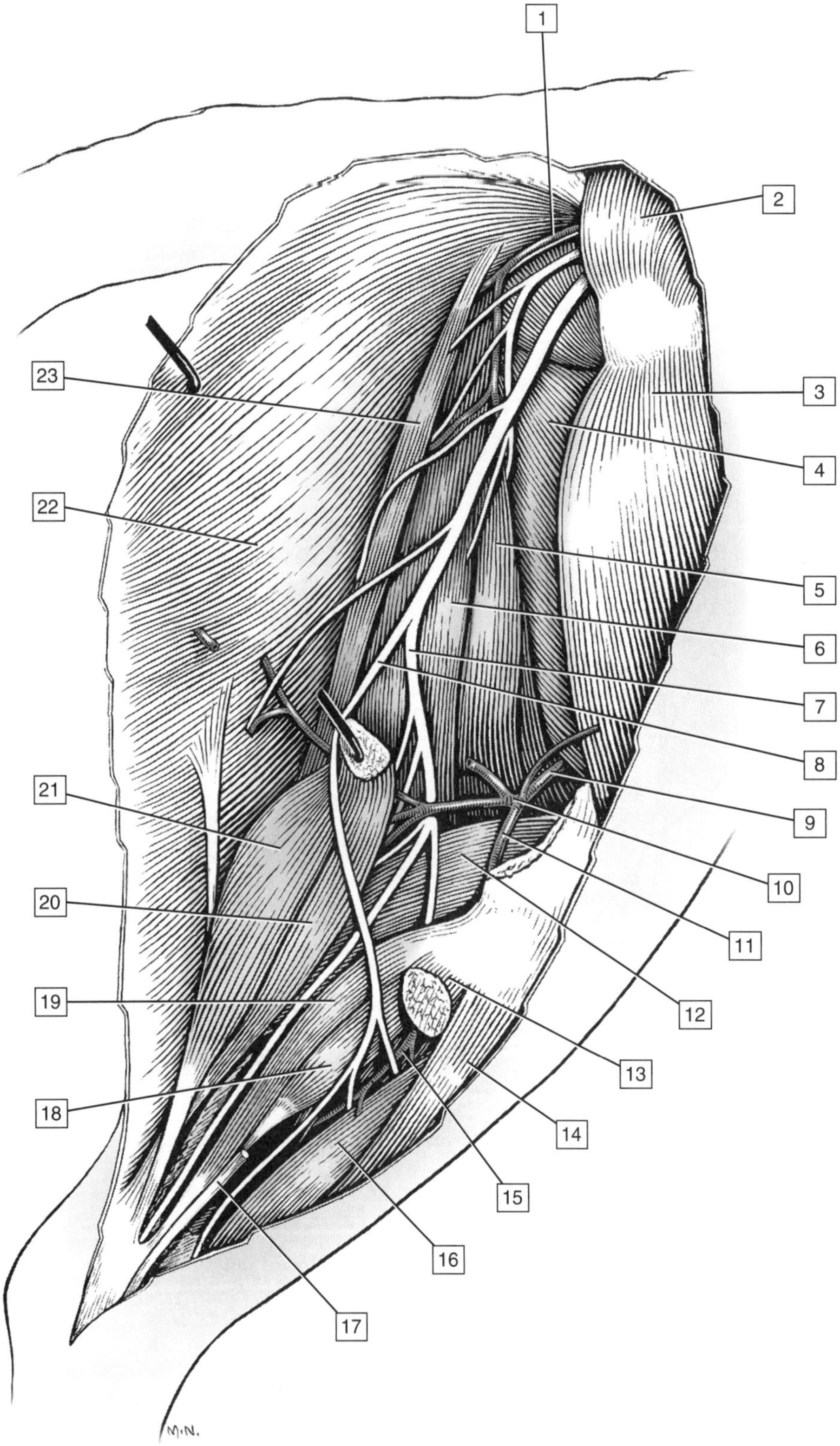

1 Caudal gluteal a.

2 Superficial gluteal

3 Vastus lateralis

4 Adductor

5 Semimembranosus

6 Semitendinosus

7 Tibial n.

8 Common peroneal n.

9 Femoral a.

10 Distal caudal femoral a.

11 Popliteal a.

12 Gastrocnemius, medial head

13 Peroneus longus (muscle transected)

14 Cranial tibial muscle

15 Cranial tibial a.

16 Long digital extensor

17 Peroneus longus (tendon transected)

18 Lateral digital extensor

19 Lateral digital flexor

20 Superficial digital flexor

21 Gastrocnemius, lateral head

22 Biceps femoris (reflected)

23 Caudal crural abductor

Figure 7-11 Cranial and lateral views of equine left femur

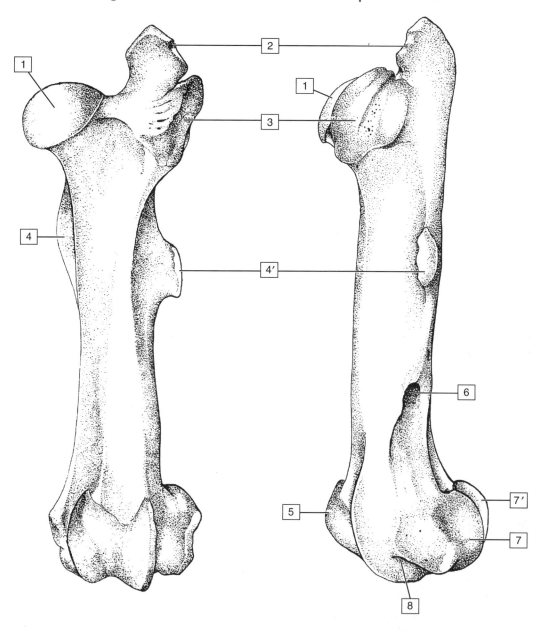

1	Head	5	Enlarged proximal end of medial trochlear ridge
2	Cranial part of greater trochanter	6	Supracondylar fossa
3	Caudal part of greater trochanter	7	Lateral condyle
4	Lesser trochanter	7'	Medial condyle
4'	Third trochanter	8	Extensor fossa

Figure 7-12   Cranial and lateral views of equine left tibia and fibula

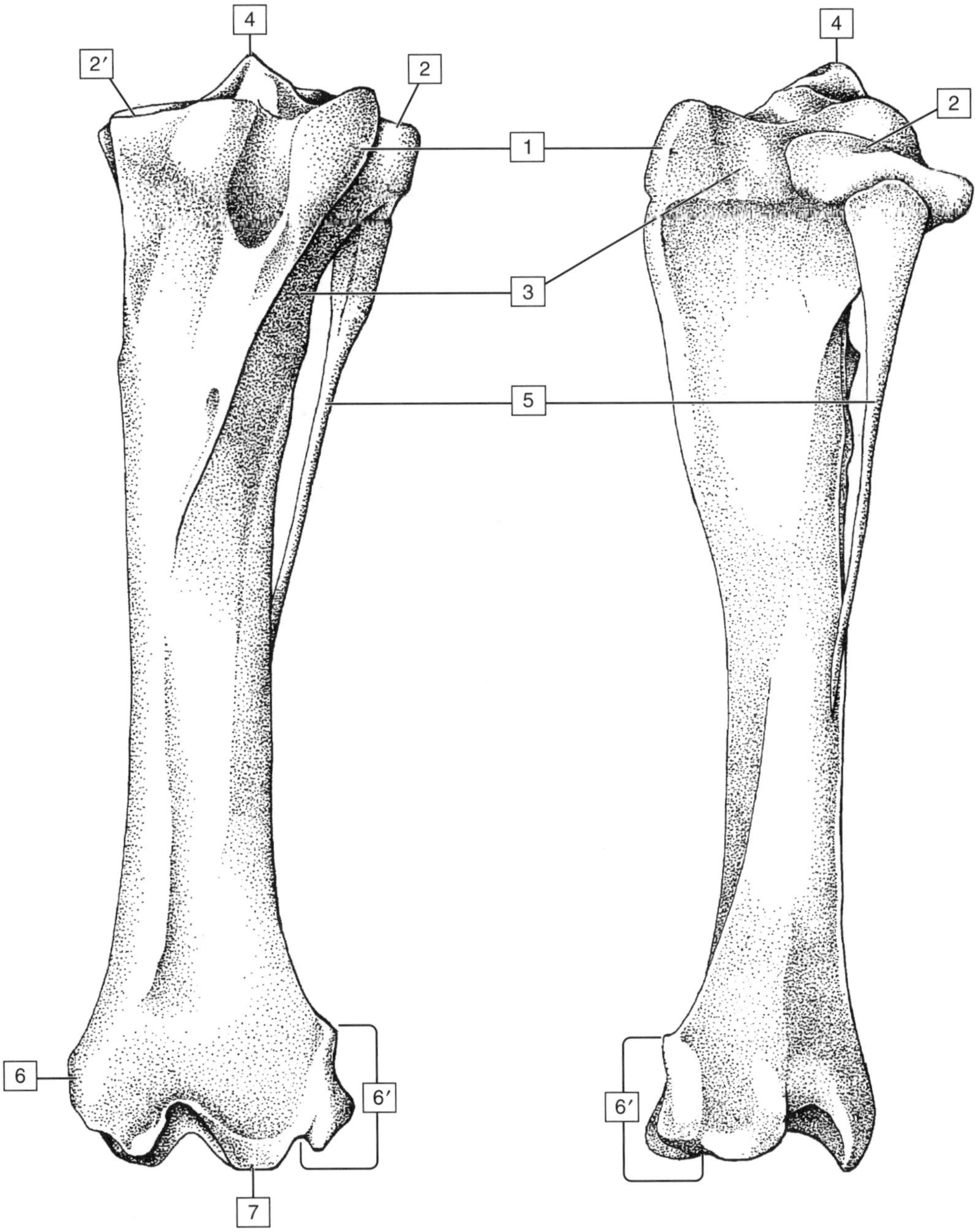

1	Tibial tuberosity	5	Fibula

2	Lateral condyle	6	Medial malleolus

2'	Medial condyle	6'	Lateral malleolus in the horse (representing distal end of fibula)

3	Extensor groove	7	Cochlea

4	Intercondylar eminence		

Figure 7-13   Skeleton of the equine left hindlimb, lateral view

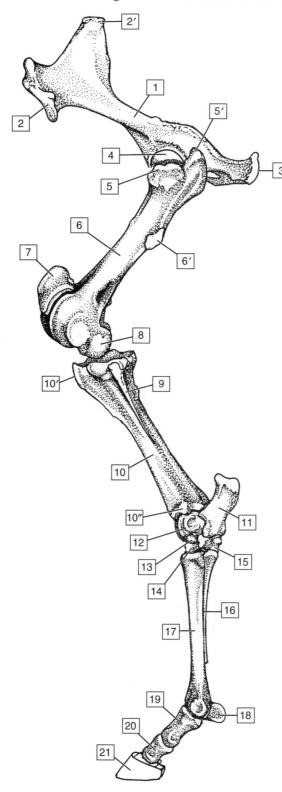

1	Hip bone (os coxae)
2	Coxal tuber
2′	Sacral tuber
3	Ischial tuber
4	Head of femur
5	Cranial part of greater trochanter
5′	Caudal part of greater trochanter
6	Femur
6′	Third trochanter
7	Patella
8	Femoral condyle
9	Fibula
10	Tibia
10′	Tibial tuberosity
10″	Lateral malleolus
11	Calcaneus
12	Talus
13	Central tarsal
14	Third tarsal
15	Fourth tarsal
16	Metatarsal IV (lateral splint bone)
17	Metatarsal III (cannon bone)
18	Proximal sesamoid bones
19	Proximal phalanx, the last within the hoof
20	Middle phalanx, the last within the hoof
21	Distal phalanx, within the hoof

Figure 7-14   Muscles of the equine thigh, medial view

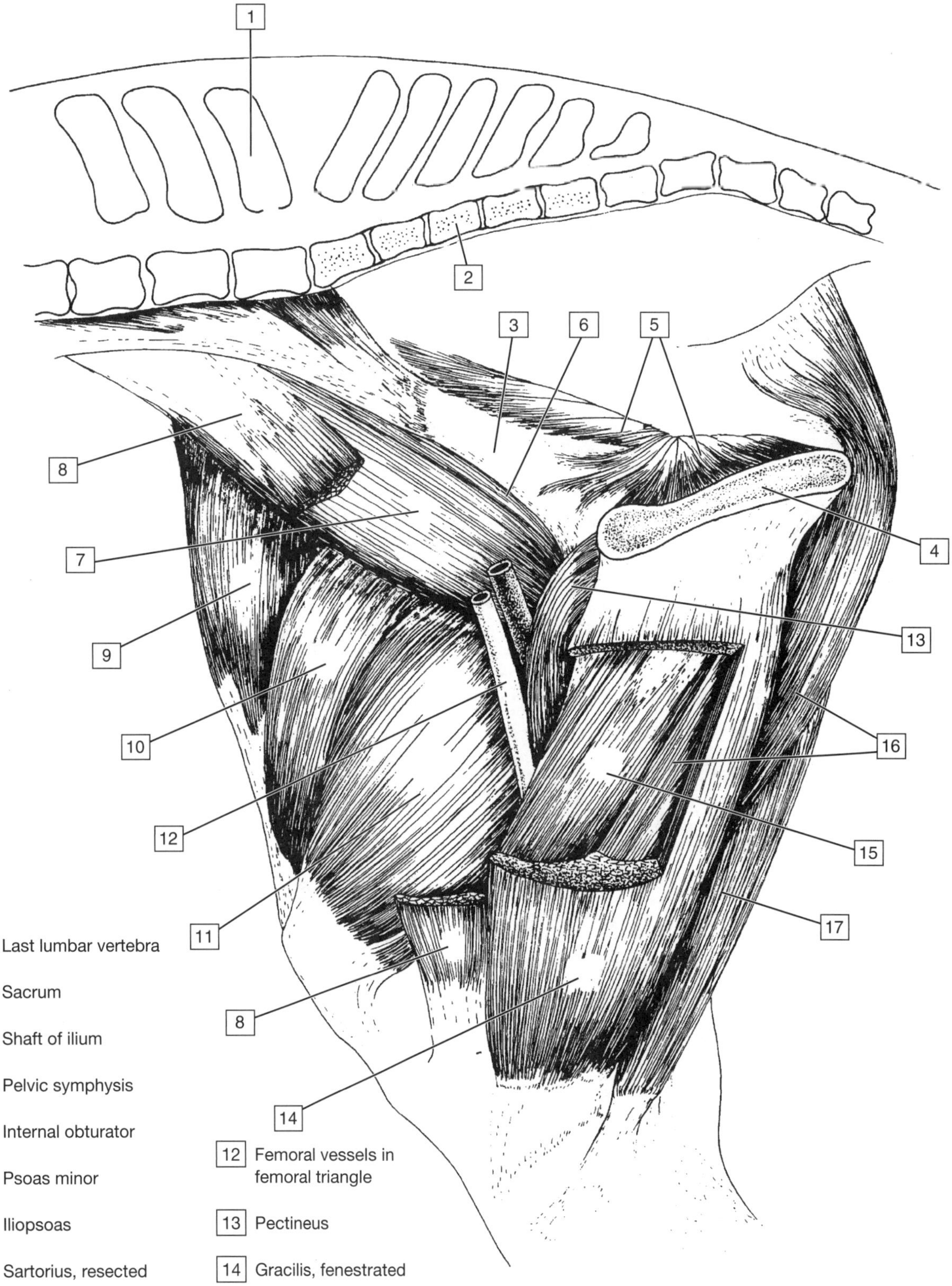

1 Last lumbar vertebra

2 Sacrum

3 Shaft of ilium

4 Pelvic symphysis

5 Internal obturator

6 Psoas minor

7 Iliopsoas

8 Sartorius, resected

9 Tensor fasciae latae

10 Rectus femoris

11 Vastus medialis

12 Femoral vessels in femoral triangle

13 Pectineus

14 Gracilis, fenestrated

15 Adductor

16 Semimembranosus

17 Semitendinosus

Saunders Veterinary Anatomy Coloring Book
Copyright © 2011 by Saunders, an imprint of Elsevier Inc.

Figure 7-15   Equine left stifle joint, cranial view

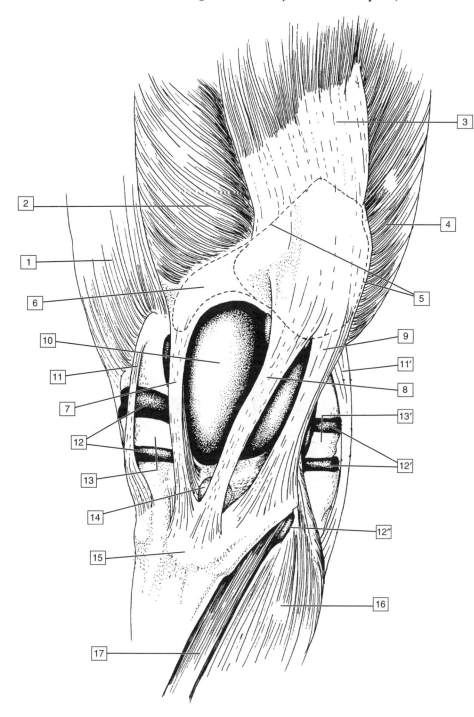

1	Adductor
2	Vastus medialis
3	Rectus femoris
4	Vastus lateralis
5	Outline of patella
6	Outline of patellar fibrocartilage
7	Medial patellar ligament
8	Intermediate patellar ligament
9	Lateral patellar ligament
10	Joint capsule over medial ridge of femoral trochlea
11	Medial collateral ligament
11'	Lateral collateral ligament
12	Medial femorotibial joint capsule
12'	Lateral femorotibial joint capsule
12"	Recess of 12' under combined tendon of peroneus tertius and long digital extensor
13	Medial meniscus
13'	Lateral meniscus
14	Distal infrapatellar bursa
15	Tibial tuberosity
16	Long digital extensor
17	Tibialis cranialis

Figure 7-16   Bursae, tendon sheaths, and joint pouches of the equine left hock

Proximal surface of a transection.

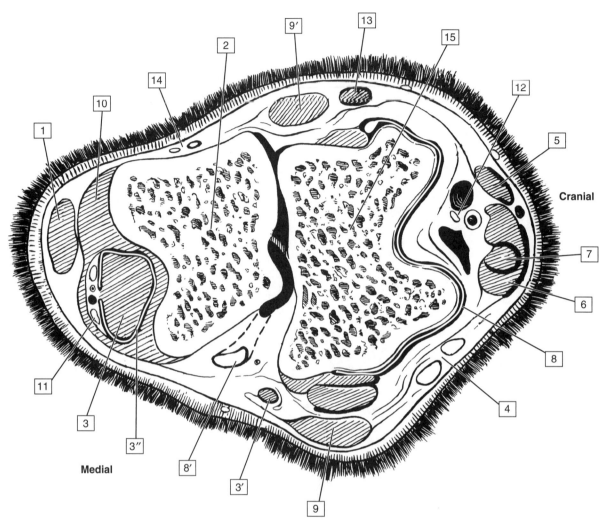

1 Superficial digital flexor	6 Peroneus tertius	10 Long plantar ligament
2 Calcaneus	7 Tibialis cranialis	11 Plantar nerves and saphenous vessels
3 Lateral deep digital flexor and tibialis caudalis tendons	8 Dorsal and medioplantar pouches of tarsocrural joint	12 Cranial tibial vessels and deep peroneal nerve
3' Tendon of medial deep digital flexor	8' Medioplantar pouch of tarsocrural joint	13 Lateral digital extensor
3" Tarsal sheath	9 Medial collateral ligament (superficial part)	14 Caudal cutaneous sural nerve and lateral saphenous vein
4 Cranial branch of medial saphenous vein	9' Lateral collateral ligament (superficial part)	15 Talus
5 Long digital extensor		

Saunders Veterinary Anatomy Coloring Book

Figure 7-17 Principal arteries of the equine right hindlimb,
caudal view

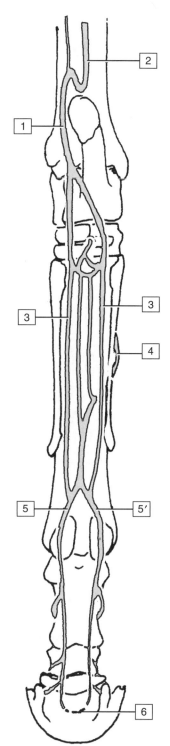

1	Saphenous a.
2	Caudal tibial a.
3	Medial plantar aa.
4	Dorsal metatarsal a.
5	Medial digital a.
5′	Lateral digital a.
6	Terminal arch, anastomosis of digital arteries within the distal phalanx

Figure 7-18   Nerves of the equine right hind foot

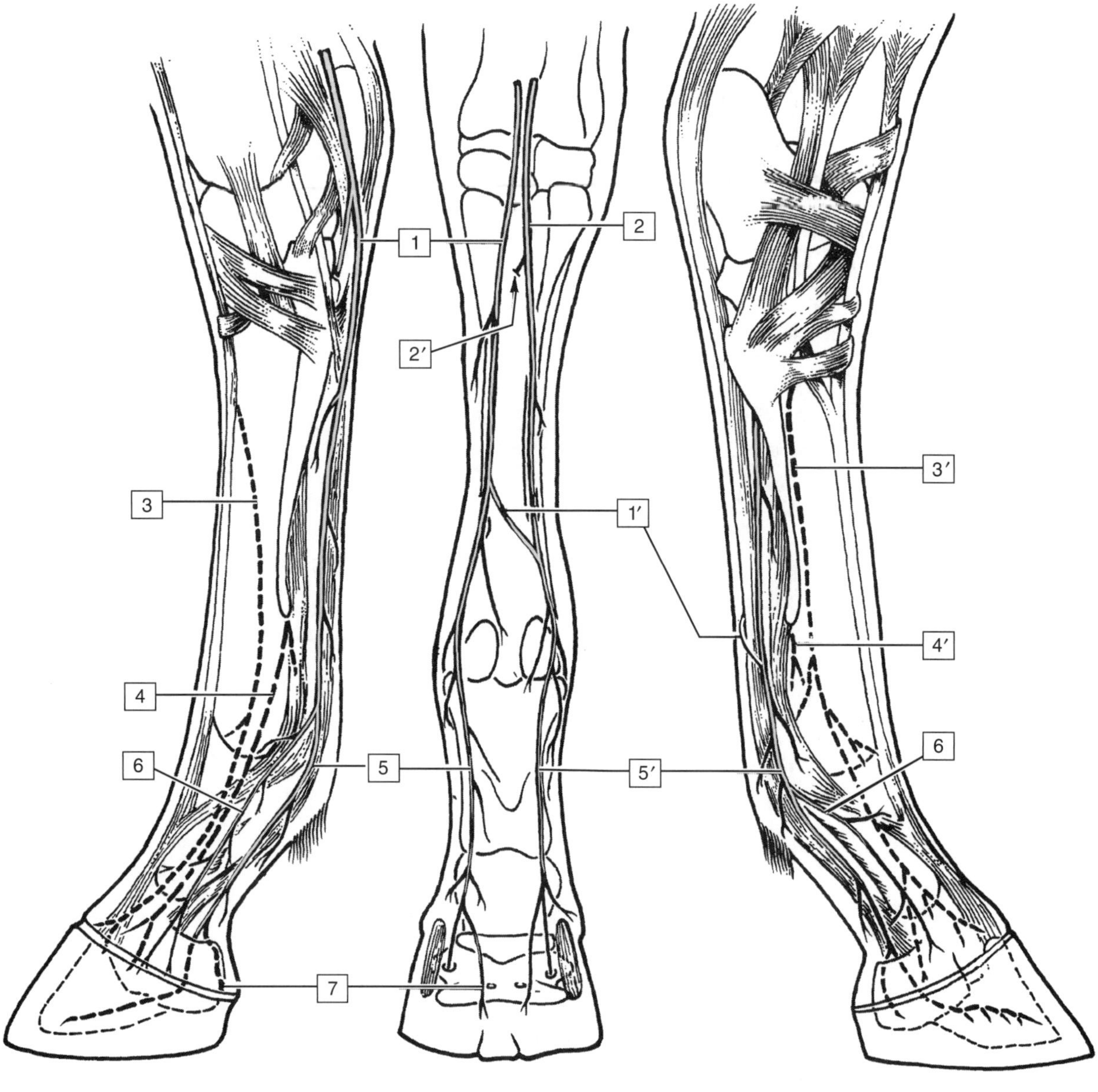

Medial   **Lateral**   **Plantar**

| 1 | Medial plantar n. (from tibial) | | 4 | Medial plantar metatarsal n. (from lateral plantar) |

1 Medial plantar n. (from tibial)

1′ Communicating branch

2 Lateral plantar n. (from tibial)

2′ Deep branch (for plantar metatarsal nn.), cut

3 Medial dorsal metatarsal n. (from deep peroneal)

3′ Lateral dorsal metatarsal n. (from deep peroneal)

4 Medial plantar metatarsal n. (from lateral plantar)

4′ Lateral plantar metatarsal n. (from lateral plantar)

5 Medial digital n.

5′ Lateral digital n.

6 Dorsal branch of digital n.

7 Branch to digital cushion

Figure 7-19   Bovine sacrosciatic ligament, left lateral view

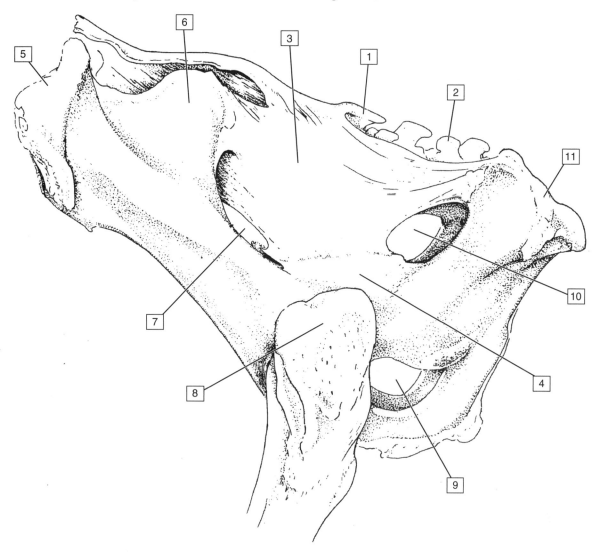

1	Sacrum	7	Greater sciatic foramen
2	Caudal vertebra(e)	8	Greater trochanter
3	Sacrosciatic ligament	9	Obturator foramen
4	Ischial spine	10	Lesser sciatic foramen
5	Coxal tuber	11	Ischial tuber
6	Sacral tuber		

Figure 7-20   Muscles of the bovine left hindlimb, lateral view

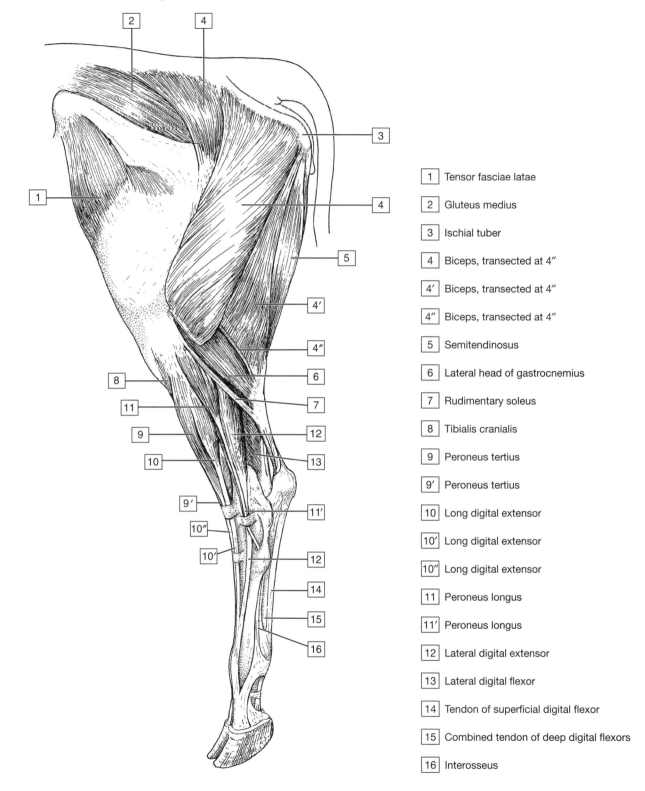

1	Tensor fasciae latae
2	Gluteus medius
3	Ischial tuber
4	Biceps, transected at 4″
4′	Biceps, transected at 4″
4″	Biceps, transected at 4″
5	Semitendinosus
6	Lateral head of gastrocnemius
7	Rudimentary soleus
8	Tibialis cranialis
9	Peroneus tertius
9′	Peroneus tertius
10	Long digital extensor
10′	Long digital extensor
10″	Long digital extensor
11	Peroneus longus
11′	Peroneus longus
12	Lateral digital extensor
13	Lateral digital flexor
14	Tendon of superficial digital flexor
15	Combined tendon of deep digital flexors
16	Interosseus

Figure 7-21   Transverse section of the bovine left leg

Medial

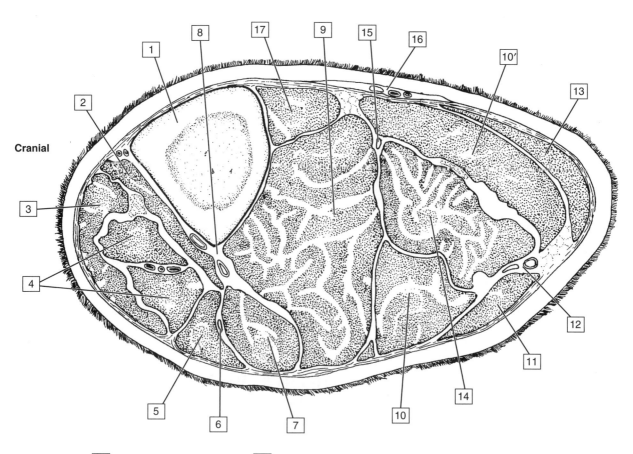

Cranial

1	Tibia	10	Lateral head of gastrocnemius
2	Tibialis cranialis	10′	Medial head of gastrocnemius
3	Peroneus tertius	11	Biceps
4	Long digital extensor	12	Caudal cutaneous sural nerve and lateral saphenous vein
5	Peroneus longus	13	Semitendinosus
6	Peroneal nerve	14	Superficial digital flexor
7	Lateral digital extensor	15	Tibial nerve
8	Cranial tibial vessels	16	Saphenous vessels and nerve
9	Deep digital flexors	17	Popliteus

Figure 7-22   Major veins of the bovine hindlimb

(A) Right hind foot, dorsolateral view. (B) Left hind foot, dorsomedial view.

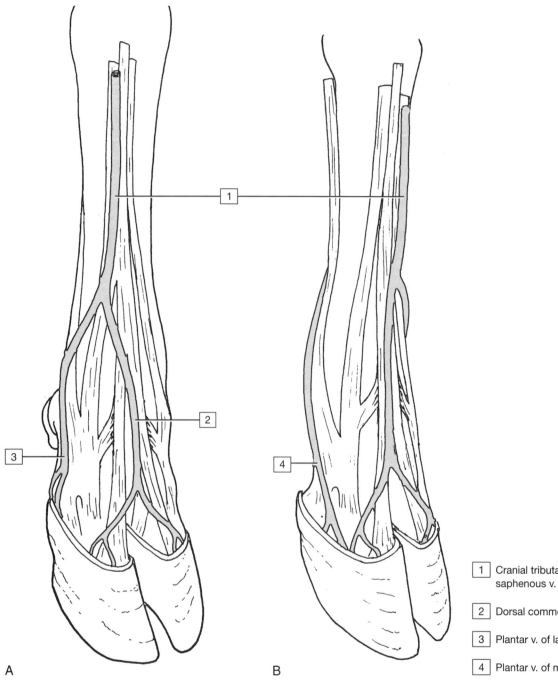

1 Cranial tributary of lateral saphenous v.

2 Dorsal common digital v. III

3 Plantar v. of lateral digit

4 Plantar v. of medial digits

A

B

Figure 7-23   Nerves of the bovine right hindlimb

(A) Right hind foot, dorsolateral view. (B) Right hind foot, plantar view.

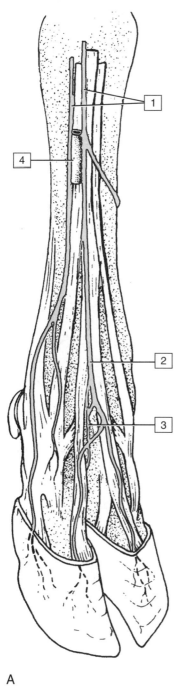

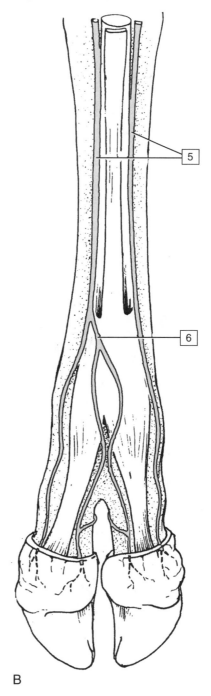

A

B

1	Lateral and middle branches of superficial peroneal n.	4	Cranial tributary of lateral saphenous vein
2	Dorsal common digital n. III	5	Medial and lateral plantar nn.
3	Deep peroneal n.	6	Plantar common digital n. III

Figure 7-24   Transverse section of the bovine left cannon

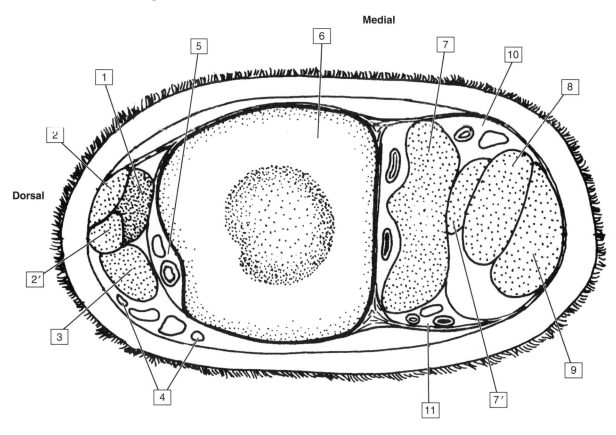

1	Extensor brevis	7	Interosseus
2	Long digital extensor	7′	Band from interosseus to superficial digital flexor
2′	Long digital extensor	8	Deep digital flexor
3	Lateral digital extensor	9	Superficial digital flexor
4	Branches of superficial peroneal nerve and cranial tributary of lateral saphenous vein	10	Medial plantar nerve and vessels
5	Deep peroneal nerve and dorsal metatarsal artery (continuation of cranial tibial)	11	Lateral plantar nerve and vessels
6	Metatarsal bone		

Figure 7-25   Lymph flow of the porcine hindlimb, lateral view

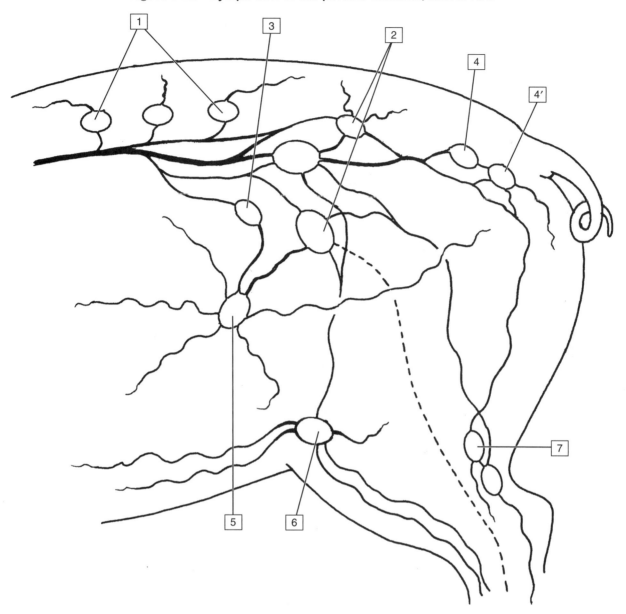

1 Lumbar aortic nodes	4′ Gluteal nodes
2 Medial iliac nodes	5 Subiliac nodes
3 Lateral iliac node	6 Superficial inguinal nodes
4 Ischial node	7 Popliteal nodes

Figure 7-26   Bones of the tarsal skeleton

Carnivores (*Car*), horse (*eq*), cattle (*bo*), and pig (*su*), schematic.
Roman numerals identify the metatarsal bones. Arabic numerals identify the
distal tarsal bones.

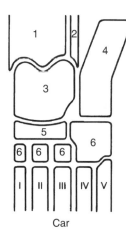

Car

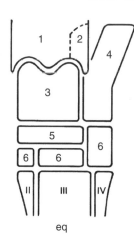

eq

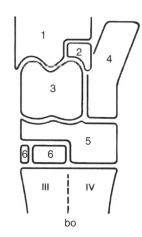

bo

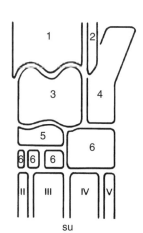

su

1	Tibia	4	Calcaneus
2	Fibula	5	Central tarsal bone
3	Talus	6	Distal tarsal bones